Cerebrovascular chronicles (stroke)

Understanding and conquering the hidden battles within

RAPHEL BOWSTON

Table Of Content

Introduction

Cerebrovascular disease, a broad term encompassing conditions that affect blood vessels supplying the brain, is a significant public health concern. It primarily includes two major categories: ischemic and hemorrhagic strokes. Here is a short story on cerebrovascular diseases. In the quiet town of Willowbrook, nestled beneath a canopy of ancient oaks, lived Sarah, a vibrant woman in her early sixties. She was known for her love of gardening, hosting Sunday brunches for her family, and her ceaseless passion for life. Sarah had always been the heart of her family, but one fateful morning, her world was suddenly cast into shadow.

It was an ordinary day, with the sun casting dappled patterns on her garden as she tended to her beloved roses. But as Sarah bent down to pluck a stubborn weed, an unexpected sensation seized her. A momentary dizziness, accompanied by an alarming numbness in her left arm, sent shockwaves of fear through her body. She tried to speak, but her words emerged as a garbled murmur.

Panicked, Sarah's mind raced. She knew something was terribly wrong. Summoning the last ounces of her strength, she staggered toward the house, each step a monumental effort. She had seen the warning signs, had heard of strokes before, but never thought it could happen to her.

Sarah's husband, David, was in the kitchen preparing breakfast. When he heard her shuffling footsteps and the incoherent sounds emanating from the hallway, he rushed to her side. The look of terror in her eyes told him that this was more than just a passing discomfort. He grabbed the phone and dialed 911 as Sarah slumped onto a chair, her face contorted with confusion and fear.

Minutes felt like hours as they waited for the paramedics to arrive. David held Sarah's trembling hand, praying for help to come swiftly. When the ambulance finally pulled into their driveway, it was a race against time to get Sarah to the hospital.

The emergency room buzzed with activity as doctors and nurses surrounded Sarah, running a battery of tests and scans. The diagnosis was grim: Sarah had suffered an ischemic stroke, caused by a blood clot that had blocked an artery in her brain. The minutes that had ticked by since the onset of her symptoms were critical, and the damage to her brain was irreversible.

Sarah's life was forever changed that day. The stroke left her with partial paralysis on her left side and difficulty speaking. Her once vibrant garden became a symbol of the life she had lost, a place of solitude where she often sat, reflecting on the fragility of existence.

This is the story of Sarah, a woman whose life was irrevocably altered by cerebrovascular disease. But it is also a story of individuals and their loved ones.

Dealing with stroke

Chapter 1

Understanding Cerebrovascular diseases

Cerebrovascular: Exploring the Vascular System of the Brain

Cerebrovascular pertains to the intricate network of blood vessels responsible for supplying the brain with oxygen and nutrients. This vascular system is essential for the brain's function and any disruption to it can have serious consequences. In this discussion, we'll delve into the importance of the cerebrovascular system, common conditions affecting it, and the significance of maintaining its health.

The Brain's Vascular Network:

The brain, despite being only about 2% of the body's weight, receives approximately 15% of its blood supply. This emphasizes the exceptional metabolic demands of the brain and the critical role of the cerebrovascular system in meeting those demands. The vascular network in the brain comprises a series of arteries, veins, and capillaries that transport blood to and from this vital organ.

The Importance of Cerebrovascular Health:

Maintaining the health of the cerebrovascular system is paramount. Any compromise in blood flow to the brain can result in severe consequences, such as strokes or other neurological disorders. To grasp the significance of this system, it's crucial to understand its role in supplying the brain with essential nutrients and oxygen.

Conditions Affecting the Cerebrovascular System:

Several conditions can disrupt the proper function of the cerebrovascular system. These conditions can be broadly categorized into two main types:

Ischemic Conditions:

These conditions involve a reduction or blockage of blood flow to the brain. The most common example is an ischemic stroke, which occurs when a clot or plaque narrows or blocks an artery supplying blood to the brain. This can result in brain cell damage or death due to the lack of oxygen and nutrients.

Hemorrhagic Conditions:

Hemorrhagic conditions, on the other hand, involve bleeding within the brain or its surrounding structures. Hemorrhagic strokes occur when a blood vessel ruptures, leading to the release of blood into the brain tissue. This can cause increased pressure and damage to brain cells.

Risk Factors for Cerebrovascular Conditions:

Understanding the risk factors associated with cerebrovascular conditions is essential for prevention. Some common risk factors include:

Hypertension (High Blood Pressure): Elevated blood pressure can weaken and damage blood vessel walls, increasing the risk of both ischemic and hemorrhagic strokes.

Smoking: Tobacco use is a significant risk factor as it promotes the development of atherosclerosis (narrowing and hardening of arteries), which can lead to blockages.

Diabetes: Poorly managed diabetes can damage blood vessels throughout the body, including those in the brain.

High Cholesterol: Elevated cholesterol levels can contribute to the buildup of plaque in arteries, increasing the risk of ischemic strokes.

Obesity: Being overweight or obese is associated with a higher likelihood of developing risk factors such as high blood pressure and diabetes.

Maintaining Cerebrovascular Health:

Preserving cerebrovascular health is crucial for overall well-being. Some key strategies to maintain cerebrovascular health include:

Regular Exercise: Physical activity promotes healthy blood vessels and helps control risk factors like high blood pressure and obesity.

Balanced Diet: A diet rich in fruits, vegetables, whole grains, and lean proteins can help control cholesterol levels and maintain a healthy weight.

Blood Pressure Management: Regular monitoring and management of blood pressure are essential, often requiring medication for those with hypertension.

Smoking Cessation: Quitting smoking can significantly reduce the risk of cerebrovascular conditions.

Diabetes Control: Managing blood sugar levels is vital for individuals with diabetes to prevent vascular damage.

In conclusion, the cerebrovascular system is a critical component of overall health, as it ensures the brain receives the necessary oxygen and nutrients for optimal functioning. Understanding the importance of cerebrovascular health and adopting a healthy lifestyle that includes regular exercise, a balanced diet, and risk factor management can significantly reduce the risk of cerebrovascular conditions and their potentially devastating consequences. It's a reminder that taking care of our vascular system is taking care of our most vital organ: the brain.

Understanding the Brain and Its Blood Supply

The human brain is a marvel of nature, a complex organ that governs our thoughts, emotions, memories, and bodily functions. While its capabilities are awe-inspiring, the brain's functioning is critically dependent on a constant and precise blood supply. This intricate relationship between the brain and its circulatory system is a topic of immense scientific interest and medical importance.

The Brain's Demand for Oxygen and Nutrients

The brain is an energy-hungry organ, accounting for about 20% of the body's total energy consumption. Despite comprising only 2% of our body's weight, the brain consumes a significant portion of our daily caloric intake. This high energy demand is primarily due to the brain's need for a constant supply of oxygen and nutrients.

Oxygen is vital for the brain's survival, as even a brief interruption in its supply can lead to severe consequences. Brain cells, or neurons, are incredibly sensitive to changes in oxygen levels. Within seconds of oxygen deprivation, neurons can begin to malfunction and die. This sensitivity highlights the brain's dependence on a steady flow of oxygen-rich blood.

The Blood-Brain Barrier

To maintain a stable and optimal environment for the brain, the body has developed a protective mechanism called the blood-brain barrier (BBB). This selective barrier is formed by specialized cells lining the blood vessels in the brain. It regulates the passage of substances between the bloodstream and the brain tissue.

The BBB is crucial for maintaining the brain's chemical balance. It prevents harmful substances, such as toxins and many drugs, from freely entering the brain, while allowing essential nutrients like glucose and oxygen to pass through. This selective permeability helps shield the brain from potential harm.

Cerebral Blood Flow Regulation:

The brain's blood supply is carefully regulated to meet its dynamic needs. Unlike other organs, which may experience variable blood flow, the brain requires a consistent supply of blood at all times. This regulation is achieved through a process known as autoregulation.

Autoregulation allows the brain to maintain a relatively stable blood flow, despite fluctuations in blood pressure. When blood pressure increases, the cerebral blood vessels constrict to prevent excessive blood flow, protecting the delicate neural tissue from damage. Conversely, when blood pressure decreases, these vessels dilate, ensuring a sufficient supply of oxygen and nutrients.

Cerebral blood flow is also influenced by neural activity. When specific brain regions are more active, they require more oxygen and nutrients. In response, local blood vessels dilate, increasing blood flow to those areas. This is the basis of functional magnetic resonance imaging (fMRI), a technique that measures brain activity by detecting changes in blood flow.

The Circle of Willis:

To further ensure a continuous blood supply to the brain, our circulatory system has a built-in redundancy known as the Circle of Willis. This circle is a ring of interconnected arteries at the base of the brain that provides multiple routes for blood to reach the brain. If one artery becomes blocked or compromised, blood can still flow through alternate pathways, reducing the risk of brain damage.

Vulnerable to Disease:

Despite its remarkable adaptability and protective mechanisms, the brain's blood supply can be vulnerable to diseases and conditions. Atherosclerosis, for instance, can lead to the narrowing and blockage of the arteries that supply the brain, reducing blood flow and potentially causing a stroke.

Another condition, aneurysms, involves the weakening and ballooning of blood vessel walls, which can rupture and result in severe bleeding into the brain. Both of these conditions underscore the importance of maintaining a healthy cardiovascular system to support the brain's blood supply.

In conclusion, understanding the intricate relationship between the brain and its blood supply is essential for appreciating the brain's remarkable abilities and vulnerabilities. The brain's constant demand for oxygen and nutrients, the protective blood-brain barrier, autoregulation of cerebral blood flow, and the Circle of Willis are all critical elements in ensuring that this extraordinary organ functions optimally. As we continue to unravel the mysteries of the brain, we also gain insights into how to better protect and preserve its delicate balance with the circulatory system, ultimately enhancing our understanding of human health and well-being.

Importance of Early Detection of Cerebrovascular Disease

Cerebrovascular diseases, including stroke and transient ischemic attacks (TIAs), are a major global health concern, often resulting in severe disability and even death. However, many of these devastating outcomes can be prevented through early detection and proactive measures. In this article, we will explore the importance of early detection and prevention of cerebrovascular diseases, along with strategies to mitigate their risk.

Cerebrovascular diseases primarily affect the blood vessels supplying the brain. The most common type is ischemic stroke, which occurs when a blood clot blocks an artery, cutting off the blood supply to a part of the brain. Another type is hemorrhagic stroke, caused by a blood vessel rupture. TIAs, often referred to as "mini-strokes," are brief episodes of stroke-like symptoms caused by temporary disruptions in blood flow to the brain. Early detection of these conditions is crucial because they can lead to permanent brain damage if left untreated.

Early detection begins with recognizing the warning signs of a cerebrovascular event. The acronym FAST is a simple and effective tool for this purpose:

F: Face drooping - If one side of the face droops or is numb, it may indicate a stroke.

A: Arm weakness - Inability to lift both arms equally or arm numbness can be a sign.

S: Speech difficulty - Slurred speech or difficulty speaking clearly is a common symptom.

T: Time to call 911 - Time is of the essence in stroke treatment; call for emergency assistance immediately if you or someone else exhibits these signs.

Beyond FAST, sudden severe headaches, vision problems, dizziness, and loss of balance can also be warning signs. Recognizing these symptoms and acting promptly can be a lifesaver.

Early detection relies not only on recognizing symptoms but also on regular health check-ups. Routine blood pressure monitoring is especially important because high blood pressure is a significant risk factor for cerebrovascular diseases. Additionally, healthcare providers may recommend tests such as carotid ultrasound to assess the health of the carotid arteries, which supply blood to the brain.

Preventing cerebrovascular diseases is equally vital.

In conclusion, early detection and prevention are paramount in the fight against cerebrovascular diseases. Looking towards the signs and seeking effective medical attention can prevent death. Moreover, managing risk factors through lifestyle changes and medical interventions can significantly reduce the incidence of these debilitating conditions. It is imperative that individuals and healthcare professionals work together to promote awareness and implement preventive measures to combat cerebrovascular diseases effectively.

Chapter 2

Types of cerebrovascular diseases

Cerebrovascular diseases refers to a group of conditions that has effect on the blood vessels supplying the brain. These diseases can have severe and often life-altering consequences, making them a significant area of study and concern within the medical field. This article will explore various types of cerebrovascular diseases, shedding light on their causes, symptoms, and potential treatments.

Ischemic Stroke:

Ischemic strokes are the most common type of cerebrovascular disease, accounting for around 87% of all cases. They occur when a blood clot or plaque buildup blocks an artery, reducing blood flow to the brain. Symptoms include sudden numbness, weakness, confusion, trouble speaking or understanding, severe headache, and difficulty walking. Immediate treatment is crucial, often involving thrombolytic therapy or mechanical thrombectomy to dissolve or remove the clot.

Hemorrhagic Stroke:

Hemorrhagic strokes, though less frequent, are more deadly. They result from the rupture of a blood vessel in the brain, causing bleeding. High blood pressure and aneurysms are common culprits. Symptoms can include severe headaches, vomiting, seizures, and loss of consciousness. Treatment includes surgery to repair the damaged vessel and manage intracranial pressure.

Transient Ischemic Attack (TIA):

Often referred to as a "mini-stroke," TIAs are referred to as short term blockages of the blood that flow to the brain. While the symptoms are similar to an ischemic stroke, they typically resolve within 24 hours. However, TIAs are warning signs that should not be ignored, as they often precede a full-blown stroke. Management involves identifying and treating the underlying causes, such as hypertension or high cholesterol.

Cerebral Aneurysms:

A cerebral aneurysm is a weakened area in the wall of a blood vessel in the brain, leading to an abnormal bulging or ballooning. Aneurysms can rupture, causing a potentially life-threatening hemorrhagic stroke. However, they can also be treated surgically or with endovascular procedures to prevent rupture.

21

Arteriovenous Malformation (AVM):

AVM is a rare condition where arteries and veins in the brain are abnormally connected, often causing a risk of bleeding. Symptoms may include headaches, and neurological defaults .Treatment options range from surgical removal to embolization or radiosurgery, depending on the size and location of the AVM.

Cerebral Venous Sinus Thrombosis (CVST):

CVST is a rare type of stroke that occurs when a blood clot forms in the venous sinuses of the brain. This can lead to a buildup of pressure, potentially causing neurological symptoms such as seizures or altered consciousness. Treatment involves anticoagulation therapy to dissolve the clot.

MoyaMoya Disease:

This is a rare, progressive cerebrovascular disorder where the blood vessels in the brain narrow and become blocked, increasing the risk of stroke. Surgical procedures, such as bypass surgery, are often necessary to restore blood flow.

CADASIL are referred to as Cerebral Autosomal Dominant Arteriopathy with Subcortical Infarcts and Leukoencephalopathy:

CADASIL is a genetic condition that affects small blood vessels in the brain, leading to a higher risk of stroke and cognitive decline. Management typically involves addressing risk factors and symptoms, as there is currently no cure.

Posterior Reversible Encephalopathy Syndrome (PRES):

PRES is a condition characterized by temporary brain swelling typically triggered by hypertension, certain medications, or autoimmune diseases. Symptoms include headache, seizures, and altered consciousness. Prompt treatment of the underlying cause is essential for recovery.

In conclusion, cerebrovascular diseases encompass a wide spectrum of conditions, each with its unique causes, symptoms, and treatment approaches. Timely diagnosis and appropriate medical intervention are critical in managing these diseases, as they can have a profound impact on an individual's quality of life and, in severe cases, be life-threatening. Moreover, preventive measures like lifestyle changes, controlling risk factors, and regular medical check-ups play a crucial role in reducing the incidence of cerebrovascular diseases. Ongoing research in this field holds promise for more effective treatments and improved outcomes for those affected by these conditions.

Causes of cerebrovascular diseases

Cerebrovascular diseases encompass a diverse group of medical conditions that affect the blood vessels supplying the brain. These diseases often result from disruptions in blood flow, which can lead to serious neurological consequences. Understanding the various types of cerebrovascular diseases is crucial for both medical professionals and the general public, as they can have severe and sometimes life-threatening implications. In this comprehensive overview, we will explore the major types of cerebrovascular diseases, their causes, risk factors, symptoms, and potential treatments.

Ischemic Stroke: Ischemic strokes are the most common type of cerebrovascular disease, accounting for approximately 87% of all cases. They occur when a blood clot (thrombus) or an embolism (a clot that travels from elsewhere in the body) blocks one of the brain's arteries, cutting off the blood supply to a specific region of the brain. This lack of oxygen and nutrients can lead to brain cell damage or death.

Subtypes: Ischemic strokes can be further categorized into two main subtypes: thrombotic and embolic strokes.

Thrombotic strokes occur when a clot forms within a blood vessel in the brain, while embolic strokes occur when a clot travels from another part of the body to the brain.

Hemorrhagic Stroke: Hemorrhagic strokes are less common but more deadly than ischemic strokes. They result from the rupture of a blood vessel in the brain, causing blood to leak into the surrounding brain tissue. This can lead to increased intracranial pressure and damage to brain cells.

Subtypes: Hemorrhagic strokes can be divided into two subtypes: intracerebral hemorrhage (bleeding within the brain) and subarachnoid hemorrhage (bleeding in the space between the brain and the skull).

Transient Ischemic Attack (TIA): Often referred to as a "mini-stroke," a TIA is a temporary interruption of blood flow to the brain. TIAs produce stroke-like symptoms that typically resolve within 24 hours. While TIAs don't usually cause long-term damage, they are a warning sign that an impending stroke may occur and should be taken seriously.

Cerebral Aneurysm: A cerebral aneurysm is a weak spot in a blood vessel within the brain that bulges and can rupture, causing a hemorrhagic stroke. Aneurysms can be congenital or develop over time due to factors like high blood pressure, smoking, or genetic predisposition.

Arteriovenous Malformation (AVM): AVMs are abnormal tangles of blood vessels in the brain that disrupt normal blood flow. They are usually present from birth and can sometimes lead to hemorrhagic strokes if they rupture. Treatment may involve surgical removal or embolization to prevent bleeding.

Cerebral Venous Sinus Thrombosis (CVST): CVST is a rare condition where blood clots form in the brain's venous sinuses, impeding blood drainage. This can result in increased pressure within the brain and potentially lead to a stroke. CVST can be triggered by factors such as hormonal changes, certain medications, or infections.

Moyamoya Disease: This rare condition involves the narrowing or blockage of the arteries at the base of the brain, leading to reduced blood flow. "Moyamoya" means "puff of smoke" in Japanese, describing the appearance of tiny collateral blood vessels that form to compensate for the blockage. Surgical revascularization is often required.

CADASIL (Cerebral Autosomal Dominant Arteriopathy with Subcortical Infarcts and Leukoencephalopathy): This genetic disorder causes thickening of the small blood vessels in the brain, increasing the risk of stroke and cognitive decline. It is characterized by recurrent ischemic strokes.

Posterior Reversible Encephalopathy Syndrome (PRES):

PRES is a reversible condition often triggered by high blood pressure or other underlying causes. It can lead to neurological symptoms such as seizures, headaches, and visual disturbances.

Risk Factors:

Common risk factors for cerebrovascular diseases include hypertension (high blood pressure), smoking, diabetes, high cholesterol, obesity, family history, age, and certain medical conditions.

Prevention and Treatment: Prevention involves managing risk factors through lifestyle changes (e.g., quitting smoking, a healthy diet, exercise) and controlling underlying conditions. Treatment may include medications, surgery, clot-dissolving drugs (for ischemic strokes), and interventions to repair blood vessel abnormalities.

In conclusion, cerebrovascular diseases encompass a range of conditions that affect the brain's blood vessels, often leading to serious neurological consequences. Understanding these diseases, their risk factors, and treatment options is essential for early detection and prevention, as timely intervention can greatly improve outcomes for those affected by these conditions.

Effects of cerebrovascular diseases

Cerebrovascular diseases encompass a diverse group of medical conditions that affect the blood vessels supplying the brain. These diseases often result from disruptions in blood flow, which can lead to serious neurological consequences. Understanding the various types of cerebrovascular diseases is crucial for both medical professionals and the general public, as they can have severe and sometimes life-threatening implications. In this comprehensive overview, we will explore the major types of cerebrovascular diseases, their causes, risk factors, symptoms, and potential treatments.

Ischemic Stroke: Ischemic strokes are the most common type of cerebrovascular disease, accounting for approximately 87% of all cases. They occur when a blood clot (thrombus) or an embolism (a clot that travels from elsewhere in the body) blocks one of the brain's arteries, cutting off the blood supply to a specific region of the brain. This lack of oxygen and nutrients can lead to brain cell damage or death.

Subtypes: Ischemic strokes can be further categorized into two main subtypes: thrombotic and embolic strokes. Thrombotic strokes occur when a clot forms within a blood vessel in the brain, while embolic strokes occur when a clot travels from another part of the body to the brain.

Hemorrhagic Stroke: Hemorrhagic strokes are less common but more deadly than ischemic strokes. They result from the rupture of a blood vessel in the brain, causing blood to leak into the surrounding brain tissue. This can lead to increased intracranial pressure and damage to brain cells.

Subtypes: Hemorrhagic strokes can be divided into two subtypes: intracerebral hemorrhage (bleeding within the brain) and subarachnoid hemorrhage (bleeding in the space between the brain and the skull).

Transient Ischemic Attack (TIA): Often referred to as a "mini-stroke," a TIA is a temporary interruption of blood flow to the brain. TIAs produce stroke-like symptoms that typically resolve within 24 hours. While TIAs don't usually cause long-term damage, they are a warning sign that an impending stroke may occur and should be taken seriously.

Cerebral Aneurysm: A cerebral aneurysm is a weak spot in a blood vessel within the brain that bulges and can rupture, causing a hemorrhagic stroke. Aneurysms can be congenital or develop over time due to factors like high blood pressure, smoking, or genetic predisposition.

Arteriovenous Malformation (AVM): AVMs are abnormal tangles of blood vessels in the brain that disrupt normal blood flow. They are usually present from birth and can sometimes lead to hemorrhagic strokes if they rupture. Treatment may involve surgical removal or embolization to prevent bleeding.

Cerebral Venous Sinus Thrombosis (CVST): CVST is a rare condition where blood clots form in the brain's venous sinuses, impeding blood drainage. This can result in increased pressure within the brain and potentially lead to a stroke. CVST can be triggered by factors such as hormonal changes, certain medications, or infections.

Moyamoya Disease: This rare condition involves the narrowing or blockage of the arteries at the base of the brain, leading to reduced blood flow. "Moyamoya" means "puff of smoke" in Japanese, describing the appearance of tiny collateral blood vessels that form to compensate for the blockage. Surgical revascularization is often required.

CADASIL (Cerebral Autosomal Dominant Arteriopathy with Subcortical Infarcts and Leukoencephalopathy): This genetic disorder causes thickening of the small blood vessels in the brain, increasing the risk of stroke and cognitive decline. It is characterized by recurrent ischemic strokes.

Posterior Reversible Encephalopathy Syndrome (PRES): PRES is a reversible condition often triggered by high blood pressure or other underlying causes. It can lead to neurological symptoms such as seizures, headaches, and visual disturbances.

Risk Factors:

Common risk factors for cerebrovascular diseases include hypertension (high blood pressure), smoking, diabetes, high cholesterol, obesity, family history, age, and certain medical conditions.

Prevention and Treatment: Prevention involves managing risk factors through lifestyle changes (e.g., quitting smoking, a healthy diet, exercise) and controlling underlying conditions. Treatment may include medications, surgery, clot-dissolving drugs (for ischemic strokes), and interventions to repair blood vessel abnormalities.

In conclusion, cerebrovascular diseases encompass a range of conditions that affect the brain's blood vessels, often leading to serious neurological consequences. Understanding these diseases, their risk factors, and treatment options is essential for early detection and prevention, as timely intervention can greatly improve outcomes for those affected by these conditions.

Prevention of cerebrovascular diseases

Cerebrovascular diseases, encompassing conditions such as strokes and transient ischemic attacks (TIAs), are a significant public health concern worldwide. These conditions can result in severe disability or even death, making their prevention a critical aspect of healthcare. Fortunately, many of the risk factors for cerebrovascular diseases are modifiable, and adopting a comprehensive approach to prevention can significantly reduce the incidence of these devastating conditions.

Healthy Lifestyle Choices:

Maintaining a healthy lifestyle is the cornerstone of cerebrovascular disease prevention. This includes

Diet: A heart-healthy diet low in saturated fats, trans fats, cholesterol, and sodium can reduce the risk of cerebrovascular diseases. Eat more of fruits, vegetables ,lean proteins, and healthy fats.

Physical Activity: Regular exercise improves cardiovascular health and helps maintain a healthy weight.

Smoking Cessation: Smoking is a significant risk factor for cerebrovascular diseases. Quitting smoking reduces this risk significantly.

Moderate Alcohol Consumption: Excessive alcohol intake can raise blood pressure and contribute to cerebrovascular diseases. If you drink alcohol dont take it in excess

Hypertension Management:

High blood pressure (hypertension) is a leading cause of cerebrovascular diseases. Regular blood pressure checks and management through lifestyle changes and medication, if necessary, are essential.

Diabetes Control:

Uncontrolled diabetes increases the risk of stroke. Properly managing blood sugar levels through diet, exercise, and medication can reduce this risk.

Cholesterol Management:

High levels of LDL cholesterol can lead to atherosclerosis, a condition that narrows and hardens the arteries, increasing the risk of stroke. Controlling cholesterol levels through diet and medication can mitigate this risk.

Weight Management:

Obesity is a risk factor for cerebrovascular diseases. Maintaining a healthy weight through diet and exercise can lower this risk.

Atrial Fibrillation Detection and Management:

Atrial fibrillation (an irregular heart rhythm) can lead to blood clots that may cause a stroke. Detecting and managing atrial fibrillation through medication or procedures is crucial.

Healthy Diet Choices:

A diet rich in fruits, vegetables, whole grains, lean proteins, and healthy fats provides essential nutrients that support overall health and reduce the risk of cerebrovascular diseases.

Limiting Sodium Intake:

High sodium intake can raise blood pressure. Reducing salt in the diet by cooking at home and reading food labels can help control sodium intake.

Stress Reduction:

Chronic stress can contribute to hypertension and increase the risk of cerebrovascular diseases. Practicing stress-reduction techniques such as meditation, deep breathing, or yoga can be beneficial.

Regular Check-Ups:

Regular medical check-ups can help detect risk factors early and allow for timely intervention. It's essential to monitor blood pressure, cholesterol levels, and other relevant health markers.

Medication Adherence:

If prescribed medication for risk factors like hypertension, diabetes, or atrial fibrillation, it's crucial to take it as directed by a healthcare provider.

Education and Awareness:

Public education campaigns and community outreach can raise awareness about cerebrovascular disease risk factors and prevention strategies. Knowledge makes individuals to make important choices about their health.

In conclusion, preventing cerebrovascular diseases requires a multifaceted approach that addresses modifiable risk factors through lifestyle changes and medical management. Healthy living, regular medical check-ups, and adherence to prescribed treatments can significantly reduce the incidence of strokes and other cerebrovascular conditions. Public health initiatives play a crucial role in disseminating information and promoting preventive measures, ultimately leading to better outcomes for individuals and communities. It is imperative that individuals, healthcare providers, and policymakers collaborate to prioritize cerebrovascular disease prevention and reduce the burden of these conditions on society.

Dealing with stroke

Chapter 3

Clinical Presentation of Cerebrovascular diseases

Cerebrovascular diseases encompass a group of medical conditions that affect the blood vessels supplying the brain. These conditions, which often result from various risk factors and underlying health issues, can manifest in diverse clinical presentations. The two primary types of cerebrovascular diseases are ischemic strokes and hemorrhagic strokes, each with distinct symptomatology.

Ischemic strokes, accounting for the majority of cerebrovascular cases, occur when a blood clot or plaque buildup in a blood vessel reduces or completely blocks blood flow to a part of the brain. The clinical presentation of an ischemic stroke typically includes sudden weakness or numbness, frequently affecting one side of the body, including the face, arm, or leg. Individuals may experience difficulty speaking, characterized by slurred speech an inability to find words. Confusion, abrupt vision problems such as blurred vision or blindness in one or both eyes, severe headaches, and trouble walking may also occur. These symptoms collectively emphasize the urgency of seeking immediate medical attention for timely interventions.

Conversely, hemorrhagic strokes, while less common, arise from the rupture of blood vessels within the brain. The hallmark symptom of a hemorrhagic stroke is a severe headache, often described as the "worst headache of my life." Nausea, vomiting, and altered consciousness may accompany this excruciating headache. Similar to ischemic strokes, individuals may experience sudden weakness or numbness, speech difficulties, confusion, or seizures.

It's essential to note that cerebrovascular diseases can also manifest as transient ischemic attacks (TIAs), often referred to as "mini-strokes." TIAs present symptoms similar to ischemic strokes but are temporary, typically lasting only a few minutes to a few hours before resolving. However, TIAs should not be ignored, as they can serve as crucial warning signs of more severe cerebrovascular issues in the future.

Furthermore, long-term consequences of cerebrovascular diseases can result in vascular dementia, characterized by a gradual decline in cognitive function due to repeated small strokes or damage to blood vessels in the brain. Symptoms may include memory loss, impaired judgment, difficulty with reasoning, and personality changes.

In conclusion, cerebrovascular diseases encompass a spectrum of conditions, with ischemic and hemorrhagic strokes representing the most prominent subtypes. Recognizing the distinct clinical presentations of these diseases is paramount for early detection and prompt medical intervention, as timely treatment can significantly improve patient outcomes and reduce the risk of disability or death associated with these conditions.

Imaging tool for cerebrovascular diseases

These tools play a crucial role in accurately identifying the condition and determining the most appropriate treatment. Here are some key diagnostic tools commonly used in cerebrovascular testing:

Imaging Scans:

CT scan (Computed Tomography): CT scans provide detailed cross-sectional images of the brain, helping to identify bleeding, ischemic strokes, or other structural abnormalities.

MRI (Magnetic Resonance Imaging): MRIs offer high-resolution images of the brain's soft tissues, aiding in the detection of stroke-related changes.

Angiography:

CT Angiography (CTA): CTA involves the use of contrast dye and CT scanning to visualize blood vessels in the brain, identifying blockages, aneurysms, or other abnormalities.

Magnetic Resonance Angiography (MRA):

MRA uses magnetic fields and radio waves to create detailed images of blood vessels, assisting in the assessment of blood flow and vascular conditions.

Doppler Ultrasound:

Transcranial Doppler ultrasound measures blood flow velocity in the brain's arteries, helping diagnose conditions like stenosis or emboli.

Electroencephalogram (EEG):

EEG records electrical activity in the brain and is used to diagnose conditions like seizures or assess brain function after a stroke.

Lumbar Puncture:

This procedure involves collecting cerebrospinal fluid through a needle in the lower back to test for bleeding or infection.

Blood Tests:

Blood tests can help assess risk factors for cerebrovascular conditions, such as cholesterol levels, clotting disorders, or infection markers.

These diagnostic tools, when used in conjunction with a thorough clinical evaluation, help healthcare professionals accurately diagnose cerebrovascular conditions and determine the most appropriate treatment plan, whether it's medication, surgery, or rehabilitation. Early and precise diagnosis is critical for optimizing outcomes and minimizing the long-term effects of cerebrovascular disorders.

Diagnosis tools for Cerebrovascular diseases

Cerebrovascular diseases, including conditions like strokes and aneurysms, are serious medical concerns that require various diagnostic and treatment techniques. Medical science has made significant advancements in this field, and several techniques are employed for both prevention and intervention. Here are some of the key techniques used in managing cerebrovascular diseases. Diagnostic imaging includes

CT (Computed Tomography) Scans:

CT scans are often the initial diagnostic tool used to identify hemorrhagic strokes, blood vessel abnormalities, or signs of atherosclerosis in the brain's blood vessels.

MRI (Magnetic Resonance Imaging):

MRI provides detailed images of the brain and is particularly useful in identifying ischemic strokes, tumors, and aneurysms.

Angiography:

Cerebral angiography involves injecting a contrast dye into blood vessels and taking X-ray images. It is crucial for diagnosing aneurysms and vascular malformations.

Ultrasound:

Transcranial Doppler (TCD): TCD is a non-invasive ultrasound technique that assesses blood flow in the

43

brain's arteries. It's used to detect abnormal blood flow patterns and is valuable in diagnosing conditions like vasospasm after a subarachnoid hemorrhage.

Blood Tests:

Routine blood tests can help identify risk factors for cerebrovascular diseases, such as high cholesterol levels, diabetes, and clotting disorders.

Electroencephalogram (EEG):

EEG measures electrical activity in the brain and is used to diagnose conditions like seizures and monitor brain function during surgery.

Lumbar Puncture (Spinal Tap):

In cases where a subarachnoid hemorrhage is suspected, a lumbar puncture can be performed to analyze cerebrospinal fluid for signs of bleeding.

Medications:

Depending on the specific condition, medications like anticoagulants, antiplatelet drugs, and medications to control blood pressure may be prescribed to manage cerebrovascular diseases.

Surgical Interventions Includes:

Endovascular Procedures:

These minimally invasive procedures, such as angioplasty and stent placement, are used to open narrowed or blocked blood vessels in the brain.

Clipping or Coiling Aneurysms:

For aneurysms, surgical options include clipping the aneurysm to prevent bleeding or coiling it to block blood flow.

Carotid Endarterectomy:

This procedure removes plaque from the carotid artery to reduce the risk of stroke.

Thrombectomy:

For ischemic strokes caused by blood clots, thrombectomy involves removing the clot using specialized tools, often through a catheter-based approach.

Rehabilitation:

After a cerebrovascular event, rehabilitation techniques, including physical therapy, speech therapy, and occupational therapy, are vital to help patients regain lost function and independence.

Lifestyle Modifications:

Encouraging patients to make healthy lifestyle changes like quitting smoking, managing weight, controlling diabetes, and reducing stress is a key preventive technique.

Telemedicine:

Telemedicine is becoming increasingly important for remote monitoring and consultation, especially for patients at risk of cerebrovascular diseases who may need regular check-ups and medical guidance.

Genetic Testing:

Genetic testing can identify hereditary factors that increase the risk of cerebrovascular diseases. This information can guide preventive measures and screening.

Neuroprotective Agents:

Research is ongoing in the development of drugs and interventions aimed at protecting brain tissue during and after cerebrovascular events, potentially reducing long-term damage.

In summary, the techniques for cerebrovascular diseases encompass a wide range of diagnostic, treatment, and preventive approaches. Advances in medical technology and ongoing research continue to enhance our ability to detect, manage, and ultimately reduce the impact of these serious neurological conditions. Early detection and appropriate intervention are crucial for improving outcomes and minimizing disability associated with cerebrovascular diseases.

Chapter 4

Symptoms of Stroke

A stroke is a medical emergency that occurs when the blood supply to part of the brain is disrupted or reduced, leading to damage to brain cells. Recognizing the symptoms of a stroke is crucial for seeking immediate medical attention, as early intervention can minimize long-term disability or even save a life. Common stroke symptoms can be identified with the acronym FAST:

Face:

Facial drooping is a key indicator of a stroke. Tell the person to smile or laugh if a part of the face looks uneven that is a sign of stroke.

Arms:

Weakness or numbness in one arm is another symptom. Have the person raise both arms; if one arm drifts downward or is unable to be lifted, it's a concern.

Speech:

Slurred speech or difficulty speaking is a prominent sign. Ask the person to repeat a simple sentence; if their words are unclear or they can't repeat it accurately, this may indicate a stroke.

Time:

Time is of the essence in stroke care. If you observe any of these symptoms, call emergency services immediately. Stroke treatment options are time-sensitive, and the faster medical help is received, the better the chances of recovery.

In addition to the FAST acronym, there are other symptoms that may accompany a stroke, such as:

Someone beginning to experience a very destabilizing head ache, moving without coordination.

Sudden confusion, difficulty understanding speech or expressing thoughts.

Vision problems in one or both eyes, such as blurred or double vision.

It's essential to note that not all strokes present with the same symptoms, and some individuals may experience a combination of these signs. If you suspect someone is having a stroke, don't wait for the symptoms to improve. Seek immediate medical attention, as early diagnosis and treatment can significantly improve the outcome and quality of life for stroke survivors.

Diagnosis of Stroke

Diagnosing Cerebrovascular Disease:

A Comprehensive Overview Cerebrovascular diseases encompass a group of medical conditions that affect the blood vessels and blood supply to the brain. These conditions can lead to serious health consequences, including strokes, aneurysms, and vascular malformations. Timely and accurate diagnosis is paramount in managing these diseases effectively and preventing complications. This article provides a comprehensive overview of the diagnostic methods and procedures used in the diagnosis of cerebrovascular diseases.

Medical History and Physical Examination:

The diagnostic journey often begins with a thorough medical history and physical examination by a healthcare professional. Patients are asked about their symptoms, medical history, and risk factors such as hypertension, diabetes, smoking, and family history of cerebrovascular diseases. A physical examination is conducted to assess neurological signs, such as weakness, numbness, or changes in coordination.

Imaging Studies includes:

- **CT Scan (Computed Tomography):**
  Computed Tomography (CT) scans are commonly employed to detect cerebrovascular diseases. They can reveal evidence of bleeding, blood clots, or structural abnormalities in the brain. CT scans provide rapid results, making them particularly valuable in emergency situations like acute stroke.

- **MRI (Magnetic Resonance Imaging):**
  Magnetic Resonance Imaging (MRI) is another crucial imaging tool. It offers detailed images of the brain, enabling the identification of strokes, aneurysms, tumors, and other structural abnormalities. MRIs are highly effective for visualizing soft tissues and

providing insights into the blood flow within the brain.

- **CT Angiography and MR Angiography:**
These specialized scans focus on the blood vessels within the brain. CT Angiography and MR Angiography can detect abnormalities in the blood vessels, such as stenosis (narrowing), aneurysms, and arteriovenous malformations (AVMs). They are instrumental in assessing the vascular component of cerebrovascular diseases.

- **Ultrasound:**
Transcranial Doppler ultrasound or carotid ultrasound are non-invasive tests used to assess blood flow in the brain and neck arteries. They are especially valuable in diagnosing carotid artery disease and monitoring blood flow during and after surgical procedures.

- **Electroencephalogram (EEG):**
An EEG measures the electrical process in the brain. It is particularly useful in diagnosing conditions like epilepsy, which can be associated with abnormal

brain electrical patterns. EEG helps guide treatment decisions and monitor the effectiveness of medications.

- **Blood Tests:**
  Blood tests can help identify risk factors and underlying causes of cerebrovascular diseases. They may include assessments of cholesterol levels, blood glucose levels (for diabetes screening), and clotting factors. Elevated levels of certain biomarkers can suggest an increased risk of stroke.

- **Lumbar Puncture (Spinal Tap):**
  In some cases, a lumbar puncture may be performed to analyze cerebrospinal fluid (CSF). CSF analysis can detect signs of bleeding, infection, or inflammation in the central nervous system, which may be relevant to the patient's symptoms.

- **Echocardiogram:**
  If a cardiac source of emboli (clots that travel to the brain) is suspected, an echocardiogram can assess the structure and function of the heart. It can identify conditions like atrial fibrillation or heart valve abnormalities that may contribute to cerebrovascular events.

- **Neuropsychological Testing:**
  In cases where patients exhibit cognitive impairment, memory loss, or other neurological symptoms, neuropsychological testing may be recommended. This battery of tests assesses cognitive function and helps identify specific areas of impairment.

In conclusion, the diagnosis of cerebrovascular diseases relies on a multifaceted approach that combines clinical evaluation with a range of diagnostic tools and tests. The choice of diagnostic methods depends on the patient's symptoms, medical history, and the suspected underlying condition. Early and accurate diagnosis is critical to initiating appropriate treatment strategies, reducing the risk of complications, and improving the prognosis for individuals affected by these potentially life-threatening conditions

Treatment and Management of Stroke

A stroke is a medical diseases that occurs when there is a sudden discharge of blood flow to the brain. Prompt and effective treatment is crucial to minimize brain damage and improve the chances of a successful recovery. The treatment and management of stroke vary depending on the type of stroke, ischemic or hemorrhagic.

Ischemic Stroke Treatment:

Ischemic strokes are caused by a blockage or clot within a blood vessel in the brain. The primary goal of treatment for ischemic stroke is to restore blood flow to the affected area of the brain. Here are the key components of ischemic stroke treatment:

1. Intravenous Thrombolytic Therapy (tPA):

One of the most common treatments for ischemic stroke is the administration of tissue plasminogen activator (tPA). This treatment can dissolve the clot and bring back blood flow. However, it must be given within a narrow time window, usually within 4.5 hours of symptom onset. Early recognition of stroke symptoms and quick medical attention are vital.

2. Mechanical Thrombectomy:

In some cases, when the clot is large or tPA is not effective, a mechanical thrombectomy may be performed. This procedure involves using a catheter to physically clear the clot from the blocked blood vessel. Mechanical thrombectomy has shown significant success in improving outcomes for certain stroke patients.

3. Antiplatelet and Anticoagulant Medications:

To prevent further clot formation, antiplatelet drugs like aspirin or anticoagulant medications such as warfarin may be prescribed. The choice of medication depends on the underlying cause of the stroke and the patient's medical history.

4. Blood Pressure Management:

Controlling blood pressure is essential, as high blood pressure is a major risk factor for stroke. Medications may be prescribed to maintain blood pressure within a safe range and reduce the risk of recurrent strokes.

5. Cholesterol-Lowering Medications:

Statins may be prescribed to lower cholesterol levels, reducing the risk of atherosclerosis (hardening of the arteries) and future stroke.

Hemorrhagic Stroke Treatment:

Hemorrhagic strokes happens when a blood vessel in the brain ruptures, leading to bleeding. The treatment approach for hemorrhagic stroke differs from that of ischemic stroke due to the bleeding involved.

1. Surgical Intervention:

Depending on the cause and severity of the hemorrhage, surgery may be necessary. Surgical procedures may involve removing the accumulated blood, repairing damaged blood vessels, or addressing an aneurysm that caused the bleeding.

2. Blood Pressure Control:

Maintaining blood pressure within a safe range is critical to prevent further bleeding. Medications may be administered to control blood pressure.

3. Seizure Prevention:

Hemorrhagic strokes can sometimes lead to seizures. Anticonvulsant medications may be prescribed to prevent seizures and manage any seizure activity.

4. Medication Management:

Certain medications, such as blood thinners, may have contributed to the bleeding in some cases. Managing medication usage and discontinuing blood thinners is an essential aspect of treatment.

General Stroke Management:

Regardless of the type of stroke, there are common elements of stroke management that apply to both ischemic and hemorrhagic strokes:

1. Rehabilitation:

Stroke survivors often require extensive rehabilitation to regain lost skills and improve their quality of life. Rehabilitation includes physical therapy, occupational therapy, and speech therapy, depending on the individual's needs.

2. Medication Management:

In addition to medications aimed at preventing future strokes (e.g., for high blood pressure, diabetes), pain management and medications to manage complications may also be necessary.

3. Lifestyle Modifications:

Encouraging a heart-healthy lifestyle is essential for stroke prevention. This includes adopting a healthy eating balance diet

4. Support and Counseling:

Stroke can have profound emotional and psychological effects on both patients and their caregivers. Support groups, counseling, and mental health services can be invaluable in coping with these challenges.

5. Preventive Measures:

Assessing and managing risk factors such as diabetes, high blood pressure, and atrial fibrillation are essential in reducing the risk of future strokes.

In conclusion, the treatment and management of stroke require a multidisciplinary approach involving emergency medical care, medication, surgery when necessary, rehabilitation, and ongoing support. Recognizing the signs of stroke and seeking immediate medical attention is critical, as time is of the essence in minimizing the long-term effects of stroke and improving the chances of a successful recovery. Stroke treatment and management have made significant advancements in recent years, offering hope for improved outcomes and quality of life for stroke survivor

Chapter 5

Post stroke Rehabilitation

Post-stroke rehabilitation is a crucial phase in the recovery journey of individuals who have experienced a stroke, a condition that can result in varying degrees of physical, cognitive, and emotional impairments. This rehabilitation process typically begins shortly after the stroke occurs and can continue for months or even years, depending on the severity of the stroke and the individual's unique needs.

The primary goal of post-stroke rehabilitation is to help patients regain as much independence and quality of life as possible. It involves a multidisciplinary approach, with a team of healthcare professionals, including physical therapists, occupational therapists, speech therapists, and psychologists, working together to address the diverse challenges that stroke survivors may face.

Physical therapy plays a central role in rebuilding strength, mobility, and balance. Exercises are tailored to the individual's abilities and can include tasks like walking, stretching, and practicing motor skills. Occupational therapy focuses on helping patients relearn daily activities, such as dressing, eating, and bathing, to regain functional independence. Speech therapy aids those with speech or swallowing difficulties.

Additionally, cognitive rehabilitation addresses memory and cognitive impairments, while psychological support helps individuals cope with the emotional impact of stroke.

Post-stroke rehabilitation is a dynamic process, adapting to the evolving needs and progress of the patient. It requires patience, determination, and the unwavering support of both healthcare professionals and loved ones. Successful rehabilitation not only enhances physical and cognitive abilities but also offers hope, empowerment, and the opportunity for stroke survivors to rebuild their lives with newfound strength and resilience.

Physical Therapy

Physical therapy, often referred to as physiotherapy, is a healthcare profession dedicated to optimizing physical function, mobility, and well-being. It plays a pivotal role in helping individuals recover from injuries, surgeries, or conditions that impact their musculoskeletal system. Here's a closer look at the significance of physical therapy:

Physical therapists are highly trained healthcare professionals who assess a patient's physical condition, mobility, and any pain or discomfort they may be experiencing.

Treatment in physical therapy typically includes a combination of exercises, stretches, manual techniques, and modalities such as heat or cold therapy, ultrasound, or electrical stimulation. These interventions aim to alleviate pain, improve range of motion, build strength, and enhance overall physical function.

Physical therapy is valuable for a wide range of conditions, from orthopedic injuries like fractures or joint replacements to neurological disorders such as stroke or multiple sclerosis. It is also vital in the rehabilitation of athletes recovering from sports injuries.

Beyond recovery, physical therapy plays a preventive role. Therapists educate patients on proper body mechanics and exercises to reduce the risk of future injuries.

Physical therapy promotes independence and an improved quality of life. It empowers individuals to regain control over their bodies and engage in activities they may have struggled with due to pain or mobility limitations.

In summary, physical therapy is a fundamental healthcare discipline that aids in recovery, promotes physical well-being, and enhances the overall quality of life for countless individuals dealing with a range of physical challenges. Through the guidance and expertise of physical therapists, patients can embark on a path to improved health and function.

Speech Therapy

Speech therapy is a specialized field of healthcare that plays a crucial role in helping individuals of all ages overcome communication and speech-related challenges. It encompasses a wide range of disorders and conditions, including speech sound disorders, language disorders, fluency disorders like stuttering, voice disorders, and cognitive-communication disorders resulting from conditions like stroke or traumatic brain injury.

Speech therapists, also known as speech-language pathologists (SLPs), are highly trained professionals who evaluate, diagnose, and treat speech and language disorders. They employ various techniques and exercises to improve a person's ability to speak, understand, and communicate effectively. These methods can include articulation exercises, language drills, voice therapy, and fluency training.

Beyond helping individuals with communication difficulties, speech therapy can have a profound impact on their quality of life. It not only aids in clearer speech and better language skills but also boosts self-esteem and confidence. For children, early intervention through speech therapy can prevent academic challenges associated with communication disorders.

Speech therapy is a dynamic field that continually evolves through research and technology. SLPs now use advanced tools and tele practice to reach clients in remote areas. As our understanding of communication disorders deepens, speech therapy remains a vital resource for those striving to express themselves and connect with the world.

Occupational Therapy

Occupational therapy plays a crucial role in the rehabilitation and management of individuals affected by cerebrovascular diseases, such as strokes. These conditions often result in physical, cognitive, and emotional challenges that can significantly impact a person's daily life. Occupational therapists are trained to address these complex needs.

Firstly, occupational therapists assess the individual's functional limitations, taking into account their specific stroke-related impairments. They work with patients to regain independence in activities of daily living (ADLs), such as dressing, bathing, and eating. This may involve teaching adaptive techniques or providing assistive devices to make tasks easier.

Cerebrovascular diseases can also lead to cognitive deficits, including memory and problem-solving issues. Occupational therapists offer cognitive rehabilitation strategies to help patients regain cognitive function and improve their ability to perform tasks requiring mental acuity.

Furthermore, emotional and psychological challenges often arise after a stroke. Occupational therapists provide emotional support and implement strategies to enhance mental well-being.

In summary, occupational therapy is a vital component of cerebrovascular disease management. It aims to enhance the individual's overall quality of life by addressing physical, cognitive, and emotional aspects of their condition, facilitating their recovery and reintegration into daily life.

Chapter 6

Secondary Stroke Prevention

Secondary stroke prevention is a critical component of healthcare, aimed at reducing the risk of recurrent strokes in individuals who have already experienced one. Stroke, often a devastating event, can lead to long-term disability or even death. Therefore, preventing a second stroke is of paramount importance.

One of the primary strategies for secondary stroke prevention is managing underlying risk factors. Hypertension, diabetes, high cholesterol, and smoking are major contributors to stroke risk. Patients are often prescribed medications to control these conditions, advised to adopt healthier lifestyles, and encouraged to attend regular check-ups.

Antiplatelet and anticoagulant medications are also commonly used to prevent blood clots, which can cause ischemic strokes. These drugs are tailored to the specific needs of the patient based on the type of stroke they experienced and other individual factors.

Lifestyle modifications play a crucial role as well. A heart-healthy diet low in salt and saturated fats, regular exercise, and maintaining a healthy weight are emphasized. Patients are educated about the importance of limiting alcohol intake and quitting smoking.

Furthermore, addressing psychological factors such as stress and depression is essential, as these conditions can contribute to stroke risk.

In summary, secondary stroke prevention is a comprehensive approach that involves medical management, lifestyle changes, and addressing psychological factors. It plays a vital role in reducing the likelihood of recurrent strokes, improving patients' quality of life, and lessening the burden on healthcare systems.

Life style Modification

Lifestyle modification is a cornerstone of secondary stroke prevention. It empowers individuals who have experienced a stroke to take control of their health and reduce the risk of a recurrent stroke. These modifications encompass a range of habits and behaviors, from dietary changes to physical activity, stress management, and substance avoidance.

Dietary Changes:

A heart-healthy diet is crucial for secondary stroke prevention. Patients are often advised to follow the DASH

(Dietary Approaches to Stop Hypertension) diet, which emphasizes fruits, vegetables, whole grains, lean proteins, and low-fat dairy products. Reducing sodium intake is also essential because excessive salt can elevate blood pressure, a major risk factor for stroke.

Weight Management:

Maintaining a healthy weight is vital. Excess body weight increases the risk of conditions like hypertension and diabetes, both of which are stroke risk factors. A combination of a balanced diet and regular exercise can help individuals achieve and sustain a healthy weight.

Regular Physical Activity:

Exercise is a potent weapon against stroke. It improves cardiovascular health, lowers blood pressure, and helps control diabetes. Engaging in at least 150 minutes of moderate-intensity aerobic exercise or 75 minutes of vigorous-intensity exercise per week, along with muscle-strengthening activities, is recommended.

Smoking Cessation:

Smoking is a leading cause of strokes. The toxic chemicals in tobacco damage blood vessels and increase clot formation. Quitting smoking is perhaps the single most crucial lifestyle change for stroke prevention. Support groups, nicotine replacement therapy, and medications can aid in this endeavor.

Limiting Alcohol Consumption:

Excessive alcohol intake can raise blood pressure and contribute to irregular heart rhythms. Stroke survivors are advised to limit alcohol consumption to moderate levels, which is generally defined as up to one drink per day for women and up to two drinks per day for men.

Medication Adherence:

It's crucial for stroke survivors to adhere to prescribed medications, such as antiplatelet or anticoagulant drugs, to prevent blood clots and reduce the risk of ischemic strokes. Regular check-ups with healthcare providers are essential to monitor medication effectiveness and adjust treatment plans if needed.

Controlling Diabetes:

For those with diabetes, tight blood sugar control is essential. This includes monitoring blood glucose levels, following dietary guidelines, taking prescribed medications, and incorporating regular exercise.

Cholesterol Management:

High cholesterol levels can contribute to atherosclerosis, a condition where fatty deposits narrow the arteries and increase stroke risk. Medications and dietary changes to lower cholesterol are often recommended.

Education and Support:

Stroke survivors benefit from education and ongoing support to help them make and maintain lifestyle changes. Support groups, counseling, and patient education programs can provide valuable guidance and motivation.

In conclusion, lifestyle modification is a comprehensive and dynamic approach to secondary stroke prevention. It addresses modifiable risk factors and empowers individuals to take charge of their health. Stroke survivors, with the guidance of healthcare professionals, can make sustainable changes in their daily routines to significantly reduce the risk of recurrent strokes and improve their overall quality of life. These changes are not only life-saving but also life-enhancing, promoting better health and well-being beyond stroke prevention.

Surgical intervention

Stroke is a devastating medical condition that affects millions of people worldwide, causing long-term disabilities and, in many cases, death. While strokes can be caused by various factors, such as atherosclerosis, hypertension, or embolisms, they all share a commonality: the potential for recurrence. Preventing secondary strokes is crucial to improving patients' quality of life and reducing the burden on healthcare systems. Surgical intervention has emerged as a viable secondary stroke prevention strategy, offering hope to those at risk of recurrent strokes.

Understanding Stroke and Its Recurrence:

To appreciate the role of surgical intervention in secondary stroke prevention, it's essential to understand stroke and why it can recur. Strokes are primarily classified into two categories: ischemic and hemorrhagic. Ischemic strokes occur when a blood clot or plaque block a blood vessel in the brain, while hemorrhagic strokes result from the rupture of a blood vessel. Both types of strokes can lead to significant brain damage.

Recurrence of stroke is a concerning issue because individuals who have already experienced one stroke are at a higher risk of having another. Common risk factors for stroke recurrence include uncontrolled hypertension, smoking, diabetes, and high cholesterol levels. As such, secondary stroke prevention strategies aim to address these risk factors and minimize the chances of another stroke occurring.

Surgical Intervention in Secondary Stroke Prevention:

Surgical intervention can play a pivotal role in secondary stroke prevention, especially for specific patient populations and circumstances.

Carotid Endarterectomy: This surgical procedure involves the removal of plaque buildup from the carotid arteries, which are located in the neck and supply blood to the brain. Carotid endarterectomy is particularly beneficial for individuals with significant carotid artery stenosis (narrowing) as it reduces the risk of ischemic strokes associated with carotid artery disease.

Carotid Artery Stenting: In cases where carotid endarterectomy is not feasible or carries too high a risk, carotid artery stenting is an alternative. A stent is placed to keep the artery open and maintain proper blood flow to the brain, reducing the risk of stroke.

Aneurysm Clipping and Coiling: Hemorrhagic strokes can result from the rupture of cerebral aneurysms, weakened areas in the brain's blood vessels. Surgical procedures like aneurysm clipping and coiling can prevent recurrent hemorrhagic strokes by either sealing off the aneurysm or reinforcing the vessel's wall.

Patent Foramen Ovule (PFO) Closure: Some strokes are cryptogenic, meaning their exact cause is unknown. In cases where a PFO (a small hole between the heart's upper chambers) is suspected as the cause, surgical closure can prevent recurrent strokes by reducing the risk of blood clots moving from the heart down to the brain.

Challenges and Considerations:

While surgical intervention can be effective in preventing secondary strokes, it is not without challenges. Surgical procedures carry inherent risks, and the decision to proceed with surgery must be carefully weighed against the potential benefits. Additionally, patient selection, timing, and post-operative management are critical factors that influence the success of surgical intervention.

In conclusion, surgical intervention has emerged as a valuable secondary stroke prevention strategy, offering hope to individuals at risk of recurrent strokes. However, it is essential that these procedures are conducted by skilled healthcare professionals after a thorough assessment of the patient's condition and risk factors. As medical technology advances and our understanding of stroke prevention deepens, surgical interventions are likely to play an increasingly prominent role in reducing the devastating impact of stroke on individuals and their communities.

Chapter 7

Pediatric cerebrovascular Diseases

Pediatric Cerebrovascular Perinatal stroke is a term that encompasses strokes occurring in the period immediately before, during, or after birth, affecting infants in their first month of life. Although relatively rare, these events can have significant and lasting consequences on a child's health and development.

The causes of perinatal stroke can be diverse, ranging from blood clotting disorders and infections in the mother to problems with the placenta or the baby's heart. These strokes can manifest in different ways, from subtle neurological deficits to more severe impairments.

The challenges in diagnosing perinatal stroke lie in the fact that symptoms may not be immediately obvious in newborns. They can include seizures, lethargy, poor feeding, or even unexpected limb weakness. Prompt recognition and evaluation are crucial for early intervention.

Treatment approaches for perinatal stroke depend on the severity and location of the stroke. Some infants may require anticoagulant therapy to prevent further clot formation, while others might benefit from therapies such as physical, occupational, or speech therapy to address developmental issues. Long-term monitoring is often necessary to assess the child's progress and provide appropriate support.

Perinatal stroke highlights the importance of prenatal and neonatal care to identify and manage risk factors that can lead to stroke in newborns. Advances in medical research and technology continue to enhance our understanding of perinatal stroke, offering hope for improved outcomes and quality of life for affected children and their families. Diseases: Understanding and Managing a Complex Challenge

Cerebrovascular diseases, often associated with adults and the elderly, can also affect children. Pediatric cerebrovascular diseases encompass a range of conditions that affect the blood vessels in the brain of individuals under the age of 18. These conditions can be challenging to diagnose and manage due to the unique physiological characteristics of children. This article explores the different types of pediatric cerebrovascular diseases, their causes, symptoms, diagnosis, and

Stroke In children

Stroke in children, though relatively rare, is a serious and often underestimated condition within the realm of cerebrovascular diseases. While strokes are commonly associated with older adults, they can affect individuals of all ages, including infants, children, and adolescents. Understanding pediatric stroke is crucial as it presents unique challenges in terms of diagnosis, treatment, and long-term care.

Unlike adults, children may not be able to articulate their symptoms, making diagnosis a complex task. Signs of pediatric stroke can include seizures, sudden weakness or numbness on one side of the body, severe headaches, and difficulty speaking or understanding language. These symptoms often require immediate medical attention.

In children, stroke can result from conditions such as sickle cell disease, congenital heart defects, and blood disorders, as well as infections like meningitis. Neonates can experience strokes due to complications during birth.

Early intervention is paramount in managing pediatric stroke. Prompt diagnosis through imaging techniques like MRI or CT scans is essential. Treatment may involve blood-thinning medications or surgery to remove clots or repair damaged blood vessels. Rehabilitation plays a crucial role in helping children recover their lost functions, and long-term care often involves physical, occupational, and speech therapy.

The impact of stroke on a child's life can be profound, affecting their cognitive, motor, and social development. Families and healthcare providers need to work together to support these young survivors on their journey to recovery.

In conclusion, while pediatric stroke is rare, it is a significant and often overlooked component of cerebrovascular diseases. Awareness, early detection, and effective treatment are critical to mitigating its long-term effects and improving the quality of life for affected children. Continued research into the causes and treatments of pediatric stroke is essential to advance our understanding of this condition and improve outcomes for young patients.

Perinatal stroke

Perinatal stroke is a term that encompasses strokes occurring in the period immediately before, during, or after birth, affecting infants in their first month of life. Although relatively rare, these events can have significant and lasting consequences on a child's health and development.

The causes of perinatal stroke can be diverse, ranging from blood clotting disorders and infections in the mother to problems with the placenta or the baby's heart. These strokes can manifest in different ways, from subtle neurological deficits to more severe impairments.

The challenges in diagnosing perinatal stroke lie in the fact that symptoms may not be immediately obvious in newborns. They can include seizures, lethargy, poor feeding, or even unexpected limb weakness. Prompt recognition and evaluation are crucial for early intervention.

Treatment approaches for perinatal stroke depend on the severity and location of the stroke. Some infants may require anticoagulant therapy to prevent further clot formation, while others might benefit from therapies such as physical, occupational, or speech therapy to address developmental issues. Long-term monitoring is often necessary to assess the child's progress and provide appropriate support.

Perinatal stroke highlights the importance of prenatal and neonatal care to identify and manage risk factors that can lead to stroke in newborns. Advances in medical research and technology continue to enhance our understanding of perinatal stroke, offering hope for improved outcomes and quality of life for affected children and their families.

Rehabilitation in pediatric stroke

Pediatric stroke, though relatively rare, can have a profound impact on a child's life. When it occurs, the focus of care extends beyond immediate medical interventions to encompass long-term rehabilitation. Stroke rehabilitation in children is a complex and dynamic process, aiming to optimize physical, cognitive, and emotional recovery. In this essay, we will explore the various facets of pediatric stroke rehabilitation and highlight the importance of a comprehensive approach.

Pediatric stroke is a cerebrovascular event that occurs in individuals under the age of 18. Its causes can vary, from congenital conditions to acquired risk factors such as infections or trauma. Regardless of the cause, the aftermath of a stroke in a child can be devastating, affecting their motor skills, speech, cognition, and overall quality of life.

The rehabilitation journey begins with the early identification of stroke in a child. Unlike adults, children may not be able to communicate their symptoms effectively, which emphasizes the need for vigilant caregivers and healthcare providers. Once diagnosed, the first step in rehabilitation is typically acute medical management, which aims to limit further brain damage and control symptoms. Once the child's condition is stable, the focus shifts to rehabilitation.

Physical therapy plays a central role in pediatric stroke rehabilitation. Stroke often leads to muscle weakness and impaired motor function. Pediatric physical therapists use a variety of techniques and exercises to help children regain strength, improve balance, and relearn basic motor skills. Early intervention is crucial to maximizing the potential for recovery. Therapists work closely with families to design personalized exercise programs that can be continued at home.

Occupational therapy complements physical therapy by addressing a child's ability to perform daily tasks. Stroke can hinder a child's fine motor skills, making activities like dressing, feeding, and writing challenging. Occupational therapists work on improving these skills, adapting tools or techniques as needed, and enhancing a child's independence in everyday life.

Speech therapy is another vital component of pediatric stroke rehabilitation. Depending on the location of the stroke, a child may experience difficulty speaking, swallowing, or understanding language. Speech therapists employ various techniques to improve communication and ensure that children can express their needs and thoughts effectively.

Cognitive rehabilitation is equally important, especially for children who experience cognitive deficits after a stroke. Cognitive therapy focuses on memory, attention, problem-solving, and executive functioning skills. It helps children regain their cognitive abilities and adapt to any lasting cognitive challenges.

Psychological support is an often-underestimated aspect of pediatric stroke rehabilitation. Coping with the physical and emotional effects of a stroke can be overwhelming for both the child and their family. Pediatric psychologists or counselors work with the child and their caregivers to address anxiety, depression, and emotional challenges, providing a crucial support system during the recovery process.

A multidisciplinary team approach is fundamental in pediatric stroke rehabilitation. This team typically includes pediatric neurologists, physical therapists, occupational therapists, speech therapists, psychologists, and social workers. The collaboration of these experts ensures a holistic approach to care, addressing the physical, emotional, and cognitive aspects of recovery.

Rehabilitation doesn't have a fixed timeline. It's a dynamic process that evolves as the child progresses. The ultimate goal is to maximize the child's functional independence and quality of life. Depending on the severity of the stroke, rehabilitation may last for months or even years.

In conclusion, rehabilitation in pediatric stroke care is a multifaceted and dynamic process that requires a comprehensive approach. Early identification, a multidisciplinary team, and personalized therapies are crucial elements in helping children recover from the physical, cognitive, and emotional challenges posed by pediatric stroke. With the right support and interventions, children can make remarkable strides in their journey towards recovery and improved quality of life.

Chapter 8

Rare and complex disorders

Rare and complex cerebrovascular diseases represent a subset of neurological disorders that affect the blood vessels in the brain, often presenting unique challenges in diagnosis and treatment. These conditions, while infrequent, can have profound and sometimes life-threatening consequences. In this article, we will explore some of the most notable rare and complex cerebrovascular diseases, their characteristics, diagnostic methods, and treatment options.

Cerebrovascular diseases primarily encompass disorders that involve the blood vessels supplying the brain. Common conditions like ischemic stroke and intracerebral hemorrhage receive significant attention due to their prevalence, but rare cerebrovascular diseases are equally important in the realm of neurology. These conditions, while uncommon, can be devastating.

One such condition is Moyamoya disease. This rare cerebrovascular disorder is characterized by the progressive narrowing of the internal carotid arteries and the formation of abnormal blood vessels at the base of the brain. The term "Moyamoya" is derived from the Japanese word for "puff of smoke," which describes the appearance of these newly formed vessels on angiograms. Moyamoya disease can lead to recurrent strokes, transient ischemic attacks (TIAs), and cognitive decline. Its rarity poses challenges in early diagnosis, often requiring advanced imaging techniques such as magnetic resonance angiography (MRA) or cerebral angiography.

Another rare cerebrovascular disease is fibromuscular dysplasia (FMD). FMD primarily affects the medium-sized arteries, including those supplying the brain. In FMD, the arterial walls thicken and develop abnormal fibrous tissue, leading to narrowing and sometimes aneurysms. This can result in headaches, pulsatile tinnitus, and, in severe cases, stroke. Diagnosis typically involves angiography, while treatment may include angioplasty and stenting to improve blood flow.

Cerebral venous sinus thrombosis (CVST) is yet another rare but complex cerebrovascular condition. Unlike arterial diseases, CVST involves the veins that drain blood from the brain. When a clot forms in these veins, it can disrupt blood flow and lead to various neurological symptoms, including headaches, seizures, and focal deficits. Diagnosis relies on imaging, often through magnetic resonance imaging (MRI) or computed tomography (CT) scans. Treatment usually involves anticoagulation therapy to dissolve the clot and prevent further thrombosis.

Idiopathic intracranial hypertension (IIH) is a peculiar cerebrovascular condition characterized by elevated intracranial pressure without an apparent cause. It predominantly affects overweight women of childbearing age. The increased pressure can lead to debilitating headaches and, if left untreated, optic nerve damage and vision loss. Diagnosis involves lumbar puncture to measure cerebrospinal fluid pressure. Treatment may include weight management, diuretics, and sometimes surgical interventions like optic nerve sheath fenestration.

In some cases, rare cerebrovascular diseases can have a genetic component. Cerebral autosomal dominant arteriopathy with subcortical infarcts and leukoencephalopathy (CADASIL) is a prime example. CADASIL is an inherited disorder caused by mutations in the NOTCH3 gene, resulting in the degeneration of small blood vessels in the brain. This condition leads to recurrent strokes, cognitive impairment, and psychiatric symptoms. Genetic testing is crucial for diagnosis, and management typically involves risk factor modification and symptomatic treatment.

In conclusion, rare and complex cerebrovascular diseases pose distinct challenges in the field of neurology. Their infrequency often leads to delayed diagnosis and limited treatment options. However, advances in medical imaging and genetic testing have improved our ability to identify and manage these conditions. Collaborative efforts between clinicians, researchers, and patients are essential to better understand these diseases and develop more effective therapies. Increasing awareness of these rare conditions within the medical community is crucial to provide timely and appropriate care to those affected by them.

Vasculitis: inflammation of Blood vessels

Vasculitis: Unraveling the Intricacies of Vessel Inflammation

Vasculitis is a complex and often rare group of diseases characterized by inflammation of blood vessels. This condition can affect people of all ages and can manifest in various forms, each with its unique set of challenges and implications. Understanding the fundamentals of vasculitis, its diverse manifestations, diagnostic procedures, and treatment options is essential for both medical professionals and patients.

The term "vasculitis" stems from two Latin words: "vasculum" (vessel) and "itis" (inflammation). At its core, vasculitis is a disorder in which the body's immune system mistakenly attacks blood vessels, causing inflammation. This inflammation can damage the affected blood vessels, leading to a wide array of symptoms and complications.

One of the key aspects of vasculitis is its classification based on the size of the affected blood vessels. There are three main categories:

Large Vessel Vasculitis: This type primarily affects larger arteries such as the aorta and its major branches. Giant Cell Arteritis (GCA) is a well-known example. GCA predominantly impacts individuals over the age of 50 and can lead to vision problems, headaches, and even aortic aneurysms if left untreated.

Medium Vessel Vasculitis: Conditions like Polyarteritis Nodosa (PAN) and Kawasaki Disease fall into this category. PAN can affect multiple organs, including the skin, kidneys, and nerves. Kawasaki Disease, mostly affecting children, can lead to coronary artery aneurysms if not treated promptly.

Small Vessel Vasculitis: Diseases like Granulomatosis with Polyangiitis (GPA) and Microscopic Polyangiitis (MPA) fall under this category. They involve inflammation of tiny blood vessels called capillaries and can affect organs like the kidneys and lungs.

Diagnosing vasculitis is often challenging because symptoms can mimic other conditions, and it may require a combination of blood tests, imaging, and sometimes biopsy of affected tissues to confirm the diagnosis.

Moyamoya disease

Moyamoya disease is a rare and complex cerebrovascular disorder that primarily affects the arteries in the brain. The name "moyamoya" translates to "puff of smoke" in Japanese, describing the hazy appearance of the tangled blood vessels that form in the affected areas. This condition is most commonly found in East Asian populations, although it can occur worldwide.

The hallmark of Moyamoya disease is the progressive narrowing and blockage of the internal carotid arteries at the base of the brain. This constriction limits blood flow to vital regions, increasing the risk of strokes, transient ischemic attacks (TIAs), and other neurological symptoms. These symptoms can include severe headaches, seizures, weakness, and speech difficulties.

Moyamoya disease often presents in childhood, but it can also develop in adults. The exact cause remains unclear, although genetics are believed to play a role in predisposition. Treatment strategies typically focus on improving blood flow to the brain. Surgical options like bypass procedures can restore blood supply by creating new pathways for circulation.

Early diagnosis and intervention are crucial to prevent further neurological damage. The rarity and complexity of Moyamoya disease emphasize the importance of

specialized medical care and ongoing monitoring to manage this challenging condition effectively.

Chapter 9

Cognitive and emotional impact of cerebrovascular diseases

Cerebrovascular diseases, which encompass conditions like strokes and aneurysms, can have profound cognitive and emotional impacts on affected individuals. These impacts vary depending on the severity, location, and extent of the brain damage caused by the cerebrovascular event.

Cognitively, individuals who have experienced cerebrovascular diseases may encounter difficulties with memory, concentration, and problem-solving. Stroke survivors, for example, may struggle with aphasia, a condition that impairs language abilities. Additionally, vascular dementia, a cognitive decline resulting from reduced blood flow to the brain, can occur, leading to significant impairment in thinking and memory.

Emotionally, the impact can be equally challenging. Depression and anxiety are common following cerebrovascular events. This emotional distress can be attributed to both the physiological effects of brain damage and the life-altering consequences of these diseases, such as disability and changes in daily functioning.

Furthermore, the emotional toll extends to caregivers and loved ones, who often face stress and emotional strain while providing support and care. It's essential for healthcare providers to address not only the physical but also the cognitive and emotional aspects of cerebrovascular diseases through rehabilitation, counseling, and support services to improve the overall quality of life for those affected and their families.

Cognitive Changes after stroke

Cognitive changes following a stroke can be profound and vary widely based on the location, size, and severity of the brain damage. These changes often pose significant challenges for both stroke survivors and their caregivers.

Memory impairment is a common cognitive consequence of stroke. Individual may have difficulty in remembering the past . This can impact daily life, from remembering appointments to recognizing familiar faces.

Language and communication difficulties are also frequent. Aphasia, which affects the ability to speak, understand, read, or write, is a well-known consequence of stroke. It can be frustrating and isolating for both the survivor and their loved ones.

Executive function deficits can occur, affecting skills like problem-solving, planning, and decision-making. This can hinder a person's ability to manage daily tasks and make independent choices.

Attention and concentration issues are another cognitive challenge. Individuals may find it hard to stay focused, leading to difficulties with tasks that require sustained attention.

Emotional changes often accompany these cognitive shifts. Post-stroke depression and anxiety are common, impacting one's overall well-being.

Rehabilitation plays a crucial role in addressing these cognitive changes. Speech therapy, occupational therapy, and cognitive rehabilitation can help individuals regain lost abilities and develop compensatory strategies. Emotional support, both from professionals and a strong social network, is vital for managing the emotional toll of cognitive changes after a stroke.

Emotional Well Being

Emotional well-being after a stroke is a complex and crucial aspect of post-stroke recovery. A stroke, often referred to as a "brain attack," can result in physical, cognitive, and emotional challenges. Understanding and addressing emotional well-being is essential for the overall quality of life and successful rehabilitation of stroke survivors.

Immediately following a stroke, individuals may experience a range of emotions, including shock, fear, anxiety, and even depression. These emotional responses can stem from the sudden and often life-altering nature of a stroke. The extent of emotional impact can vary widely, depending on factors such as the severity of the stroke, the individual's pre-stroke mental health, and their support system.

Depression is a prevalent emotional consequence of stroke. It can hinder recovery by affecting motivation, engagement in therapy, and adherence to medication regimens. Identifying and treating post-stroke depression is crucial. This may involve counseling, medication, or a combination of both.

Anxiety is another common emotional challenge. Stroke survivors may worry about future strokes, the ability to regain independence, or changes in their relationships. Support groups and therapy can help individuals cope with anxiety and develop strategies to manage their worries.

Stroke survivors may also grapple with grief over lost abilities or changes in their life roles. Acceptance and adjustment take time, but rehabilitation and support services can facilitate this process.

Social support plays a pivotal role in emotional recovery. Family and friends can provide invaluable emotional support, reducing feelings of isolation and depression. Rehabilitation teams, including physical and occupational therapists, often incorporate emotional well-being into their care plans.

In conclusion, addressing emotional well-being after a stroke is integral to the recovery process. Stroke survivors should receive comprehensive care that considers their emotional needs alongside physical and cognitive rehabilitation. With appropriate support and intervention, many stroke survivors can experience improved emotional well-being and an enhanced quality of life. It's important to note that recovery is unique to each 0individual, and a holistic approach is essential for optimizing emotional well-being after a stroke

Battling Depression and anxiety

Combating depression and anxiety after a stroke requires a multifaceted approach that combines medical intervention, psychological support, and lifestyle changes. Here are some strategies to help address these emotional challenges:

Seek Medical Guidance: Consult a healthcare professional, such as a neurologist or psychiatrist, who specializes in stroke recovery. They can assess your condition, provide medication if necessary, and monitor your progress.

Medication: In some cases, treatment such as antidepressants or anti-anxiety drugs, may be prescribed to take care of symptoms. It's crucial to follow your doctor's recommendations and report any side effects or changes in your condition.

Psychotherapy: Cognitive-behavioral therapy (CBT) and talk therapy can be highly effective in addressing depression and anxiety. A therapist can help you identify negative thought patterns, develop coping strategies, and work through emotional challenges.

Support Groups: Joining a stroke survivor support group or a group focused on depression and anxiety can provide a sense of community and understanding. Sharing experiences with others who have faced similar challenges can be therapeutic.

Healthy Lifestyle Choices: Adopting a healthy lifestyle can significantly impact emotional well-being. Focus on:

Physical Activity: Engage in physical therapy and exercise as recommended by your healthcare team. Regular physical activity can boost mood and reduce anxiety.

Nutrition: Maintain a balanced diet rich in fruits, vegetables, lean proteins, and whole grains. Proper nutrition supports brain health and overall well-being.

Sleep: Ensure you get enough quality sleep, as sleep disturbances can exacerbate emotional issues. Establish a sleep routine and address any sleep disorders with your doctor.

Stress Reduction: Practice relaxation techniques such as mindfulness, deep breathing exercises, or meditation to manage stress.

Social Support: Stay connected with friends and family. Isolation can worsen depression and anxiety, so maintain meaningful social connections and communicate your feelings with loved ones.

Set Realistic Goals: Establish achievable goals for your recovery, both short-term and long-term. Celebrate small victories along the way to boost your self-esteem and motivation.

Stay Informed: Educate yourself about stroke recovery and emotional health. Understanding the challenges you face can help you better cope with them.

Monitor Your Progress: Keep a journal to track your emotional state, noting any triggers or patterns. Share this information with your healthcare team or therapist to adjust your treatment plan as needed.

Patience and Self-Compassion: Recovery from a stroke is a journey that takes time. Be patient with yourself and practice self-compassion. Recognize that setbacks are a natural part of the process.

Remember that depression and anxiety are treatable conditions, and recovery is possible. It's essential to collaborate closely with your healthcare team, follow their recommendations, and actively engage in your rehabilitation and emotional well-being. Seek help and support when needed, and don't hesitate to reach out to professionals and loved ones for assistance during this challenging time

Chapter 10

Global Impact and health Care policy

Stroke is a global health crisis with far-reaching impacts, necessitating comprehensive healthcare policies to address its prevention, treatment, and rehabilitation. This essay will delve into the global impact of stroke on healthcare and explore the policies needed to mitigate its effects.

Stroke is a leading cause of death and distableness worldwide, affecting billions of people each year. The World Health Organization (WHO) reports that over 15 million people suffer from stroke annually, with more than 5 million succumbing to it. The consequences of stroke extend beyond individual suffering, as it imposes a substantial burden on healthcare systems and economies.

From a healthcare perspective, stroke care is resource-intensive. It demands immediate medical attention, often involving complex diagnostic procedures like CT scans and treatments such as thrombolytic therapy. In the acute phase, rapid intervention is critical to minimizing brain damage. However, this requires well-equipped hospitals, trained medical personnel, and efficient systems for patient transportation, all of which can strain healthcare budgets.

Post-stroke care and rehabilitation further compound the healthcare challenge. Stroke survivors often face long-term physical, cognitive, and emotional impairments. Comprehensive rehabilitation services, including physical therapy, occupational therapy, and psychological support, are essential for their recovery and reintegration into society.

To address these challenges, healthcare policies should adopt a multifaceted approach:

Preventive Measures: Policies must prioritize stroke prevention through public health initiatives. Encouraging healthy lifestyles, promoting regular medical check-ups, and controlling risk factors such as hypertension, diabetes, and obesity are essential components. Governments can also implement tobacco control measures and regulate the salt content in processed foods to reduce stroke risk.

Access to Care: Healthcare policies should aim to improve access to stroke care. This involves expanding the availability of well-equipped stroke centers and ensuring that trained healthcare professionals are accessible, especially in rural and underserved areas. Telemedicine can play a pivotal role in bringing specialized stroke care to remote regions.

Emergency Response Systems: Developing efficient pre-hospital emergency response systems can significantly reduce stroke-related disabilities. Policies should focus on enhancing emergency medical services, enabling rapid diagnosis and transport of stroke patients to appropriate facilities.

Rehabilitation Services: Robust policies should ensure that rehabilitation services are readily available and affordable. This might involve increasing the number of rehabilitation centers, subsidizing rehabilitation costs, and promoting community-based rehabilitation programs.

Public Awareness and Education: Healthcare policies should support public awareness campaigns to educate individuals about stroke symptoms, risk factors, and the importance of seeking immediate medical attention. These campaigns can also emphasize the role of primary care in stroke prevention.

Research and Innovation: Governments should invest in stroke research and innovation to develop better treatments and interventions. This includes funding studies on stroke prevention, rehabilitation techniques, and medical advancements like telemedicine and wearable devices.

Health Insurance Coverage: Policies should ensure that health insurance coverage includes stroke-related treatments and rehabilitation. This will alleviate the financial burden on stroke survivors and their families.

International Cooperation: Given the global nature of stroke, international cooperation is vital. Collaborative efforts can facilitate the exchange of best practices, research findings, and resources for stroke care and prevention.

In conclusion, stroke's global impact on healthcare is undeniable, demanding a comprehensive and integrated policy approach. Prevention, access to care, emergency response, rehabilitation, public awareness, research, insurance coverage, and international cooperation are all crucial facets of a comprehensive stroke healthcare policy. By addressing stroke on these multiple fronts, healthcare systems can reduce the burden of this devastating condition and improve the quality of life for stroke survivors and their families.

Disparities in stoke care

Stroke, a sudden interruption of blood flow to the brain, is a medical emergency demanding swift and effective treatment. However, access to quality care and outcomes following a stroke are far from uniform. Disparities in stroke care have emerged as a significant challenge to achieving equity in health.

Access to Timely Care:

One glaring disparity in stroke care is access to timely treatment. In urban areas with well-equipped hospitals and specialized stroke centers, individuals who experience a stroke are more likely to receive timely interventions like thrombolytic therapy or mechanical thrombectomy. These treatments can significantly improve outcomes but are time-sensitive.

Conversely, rural or underserved areas often suffer from limited access to healthcare facilities, leading to delays in treatment. Geography can be a significant barrier, as individuals living far from a stroke center may lose precious minutes in transit. These delays can result in irreversible brain damage and poorer outcomes.

Quality of Care:

The quality of stroke care can also vary widely. Comprehensive stroke care teams, including neurologists, neurosurgeons, and rehabilitation specialists, are crucial for optimal recovery. Disparities arise when some hospitals lack the resources or expertise to provide such comprehensive care.

Moreover, the application of evidence-based stroke treatment protocols can differ. Hospitals that follow these protocols tend to offer better care and outcomes. However, not all medical facilities adhere to these standards, contributing to disparities in the quality of care received by stroke patients.

Socioeconomic Factors:

Socioeconomic status plays a significant role in disparities in stroke care. People with lower incomes or inadequate health insurance may face significant barriers in accessing necessary treatments and post-stroke rehabilitation. Financial constraints can deter individuals from seeking preventive care or addressing risk factors, such as hypertension, which can lead to strokes.

Racial and Ethnic Disparities:

Racial and ethnic disparities in stroke care are deeply concerning. Studies have consistently shown that minority populations, particularly Black and Hispanic individuals, are at a higher risk of strokes. However, they are also more likely to receive suboptimal care, resulting in worse outcomes. These disparities can be attributed to systemic racism, social determinants of health, and unequal access to healthcare services.

Addressing Disparities in Stroke Care:

Efforts to address these disparities in stroke care are multifaceted. Initiatives must focus on improving access to healthcare services in underserved areas, including telemedicine options for rural communities. Public health campaigns should prioritize stroke education, emphasizing the importance of recognizing stroke symptoms and seeking immediate medical attention.

Standardizing stroke care protocols and encouraging their implementation across all healthcare facilities can enhance the quality of care. Equitable access to rehabilitation services and support for stroke survivors is also critical in achieving better outcomes and reducing disparities.

Furthermore, addressing socioeconomic disparities and structural racism in healthcare systems is paramount. This includes expanding health insurance coverage, improving economic opportunities for marginalized communities, and dismantling systemic barriers that perpetuate inequality in care.

In conclusion, disparities in stroke care represent a substantial challenge to achieving health equity. Timely access to quality care, regardless of geographic location, socioeconomic status, or racial background, should be a fundamental right. Addressing these disparities requires a comprehensive approach that encompasses healthcare policy reform, community education, and efforts to eliminate systemic biases. By working collectively, we can strive for a future where all stroke patients have an equal chance at recovery and a better quality of life.

Advances in cerebrovascular research

Cerebrovascular research has witnessed significant advancements over the past few decades, leading to a deeper understanding of the intricate mechanisms governing the brain's blood vessels. These vessels, including arteries and veins, play a vital role in supplying the brain with oxygen and nutrients, making cerebrovascular health crucial for overall brain function. As technology has progressed and research techniques have evolved, our ability to investigate and address cerebrovascular disorders has greatly improved.

One of the most significant breakthroughs in cerebrovascular research has been the development of advanced imaging techniques. Magnetic Resonance Imaging (MRI) and Computed Tomography (CT) scans have revolutionized our ability to visualize the brain's blood vessels. These non-invasive methods provide detailed images of blood flow, helping clinicians diagnose conditions such as ischemic strokes, aneurysms, and arteriovenous malformations with remarkable precision.

Furthermore, the development of techniques like functional MRI (fMRI) has allowed researchers to study not just the structure but also the function of cerebrovascular networks. This has opened doors to understanding how blood flow patterns change during cognitive tasks, potentially leading to insights into disorders like Alzheimer's disease.

Advancements in genetics and molecular biology have also played a crucial role in cerebrovascular research. Researchers have identified various genetic factors that contribute to the risk of conditions like intracranial aneurysms and cerebral arteriovenous malformations. This knowledge is instrumental in developing personalized treatments and preventive measures for individuals with a genetic predisposition to these conditions.

In recent years, the field of cerebrovascular research has embraced the promise of regenerative medicine. Stem cell therapy and tissue engineering hold potential for repairing damaged blood vessels in the brain. While still in experimental stages, these approaches offer hope for patients with conditions like Moyamoya disease, where blood flow to the brain is severely restricted due to the narrowing of arteries.

Advancements in neurointerventional procedures have transformed the treatment landscape for cerebrovascular disorders. Techniques such as endovascular coiling and stent-assisted coiling have revolutionized the treatment of intracranial aneurysms, making surgery less invasive and more effective. Additionally, mechanical thrombectomy, a procedure used to remove blood clots in the brain's blood vessels, has revolutionized stroke care, significantly improving outcomes for patients with acute ischemic strokes.

Another promising avenue in cerebrovascular research is the exploration of neuroprotective agents. Researchers are actively investigating drugs and compounds that can protect brain cells from damage during conditions like stroke. These neuroprotective agents could potentially extend the treatment window for stroke patients, increasing their chances of a full recovery.

The importance of lifestyle factors in cerebrovascular health cannot be overstated. Research in this area has highlighted the impact of diet, exercise, and stress management on the risk of stroke and other cerebrovascular disorders. Public health campaigns and educational efforts have become more effective in promoting awareness of these modifiable risk factors, leading to healthier choices and potentially reducing the overall burden of cerebrovascular diseases.

In conclusion, cerebrovascular research has made remarkable strides in recent years, driven by advancements in imaging technology, genetics, regenerative medicine, interventional procedures, neuroprotective therapies, and lifestyle interventions. These developments have not only expanded our understanding of cerebrovascular disorders but have also transformed the way we diagnose and treat them. As we continue to delve deeper into the complexities of the brain's blood vessels, we can look forward to further breakthroughs that will improve the lives of individuals at risk of or affected by cerebrovascular diseases.

Stroke on a Global scale

Stroke is a global health crisis that transcends borders, affecting millions of people each year and burdening healthcare systems worldwide. This debilitating and often deadly condition knows no boundaries, striking individuals of all ages and backgrounds, regardless of race, gender, or socio-economic status. In this article, we delve into the sweeping impact of stroke on a global scale, exploring its causes, consequences, and the urgent need for international collaboration in combating this silent epidemic.

The Alarming Numbers:

Stroke is a leading cause of death and disability worldwide. According to the World Health Organization (WHO), it is responsible for approximately 11% of total deaths globally, with more than 6 million people dying from stroke each year. This is a staggering number, and it's compounded by the fact that millions more survivors are left with long-term disabilities, including paralysis, speech impairment, and cognitive deficits.

Geographical Disparities:

While stroke is a global problem, its prevalence and impact vary significantly by region. High-income countries generally have lower stroke rates due to better access to healthcare, education, and lifestyle factors. In contrast, low- and middle-income countries bear a disproportionately heavy burden of stroke. The reasons behind this disparity are multifaceted and include limited access to quality healthcare, a higher prevalence of risk factors such as hypertension and smoking, and inadequate public health campaigns.

The Role of Risk Factors:

Several risk factors contribute to the rising incidence of stroke worldwide. Hypertension, or high blood pressure, is the leading modifiable risk factor for stroke. As global diets shift towards processed foods and sedentary lifestyles become more common, the prevalence of hypertension has risen. Additionally, smoking, excessive alcohol consumption, poor diet, physical inactivity, and obesity are all significant contributors to the global stroke epidemic.

The Economic Burden:

The impact of stroke goes beyond its toll on human lives and health. It also places a huge economic burden on societies. The cost of treating stroke-related medical conditions, rehabilitation, and lost productivity is estimated to be in the hundreds of billions of dollars annually. This cost places a significant strain on healthcare systems and underscores the importance of prevention and early intervention.

Prevention and Awareness:

Preventing stroke on a global scale necessitates a multi-pronged approach. First and foremost, public awareness campaigns are crucial. Educating people about the risk factors for stroke and the importance of lifestyle modifications, such as a healthy diet and regular exercise, can go a long way in reducing the incidence of stroke.

Access to quality healthcare is another critical aspect. In many low- and middle-income countries, healthcare systems are underfunded and lack the necessary infrastructure to provide timely stroke care. International organizations and governments must invest in improving healthcare systems and ensuring that life-saving treatments, such as clot-busting drugs and rehabilitation services, are accessible to all.

Global Collaboration:

Stroke is not a problem that any one country can solve in isolation. It requires international collaboration among governments, healthcare organizations, and research institutions. Sharing best practices, conducting joint research, and coordinating efforts to improve stroke care and prevention are vital steps in addressing this global crisis.

In conclusion, stroke is a silent epidemic that affects millions of people around the world and places a significant burden on both individuals and societies. While stroke's impact is pervasive, it is not insurmountable. Through increased awareness, prevention efforts, and global collaboration, we can work towards reducing the prevalence of stroke and improving the quality of life for those affected by this devastating condition. The time to act is now, for stroke knows no borders, and its consequences are far-reaching

Chapter 11

Living with cerebrovascular diseases

Living with Cerebrovascular Disease: Navigating Challenges and Embracing Hope Cerebrovascular disease encompasses a range of conditions affecting the blood vessels in the brain, including strokes, aneurysms, and vascular malformations. A diagnosis of cerebrovascular disease can be life-altering, impacting every aspect of an individual's life. In this essay, we'll explore what it means to live with cerebrovascular disease, the challenges it presents, and the hope that can be found in managing this condition.

The Impact of Cerebrovascular Disease

Living with cerebrovascular disease often entails a series of physical, emotional, and lifestyle changes. Here are some of the key aspects of this experience:

Physical Challenges: Depending on the severity of the condition and the type of cerebrovascular disease, individuals may face a range of physical challenges. Stroke survivors, for example, may experience partial paralysis,

difficulty speaking, or impaired vision. Managing these physical effects can require intensive rehabilitation and ongoing medical care.

Emotional Struggles: A cerebrovascular disease diagnosis can be emotionally devastating. Coping with the sudden or gradual onset of symptoms, the fear of future complications, and the impact on one's independence can lead to anxiety, depression, or other emotional health challenges.

Lifestyle Adjustments: Lifestyle changes are often necessary to manage cerebrovascular disease. This can include dietary modifications to control blood pressure and cholesterol, regular exercise, and medication adherence. Additionally, some individuals may need to adapt their living environment to accommodate physical limitations.

Support and Coping Strategies

Despite the profound challenges associated with cerebrovascular disease, there are strategies and support systems that can help individuals lead fulfilling lives:

Medical Care: Regular medical check-ups and consultations with neurologists or vascular specialists are essential. These professionals can monitor the condition, adjust medications, and provide guidance on managing risk factors.

Rehabilitation: Physical therapy, occupational therapy, and speech therapy can be crucial for regaining function and independence after a stroke or other cerebrovascular events. These therapies aim to improve mobility, speech, and cognitive skills.

Emotional Support: Mental health is a significant component of living with cerebrovascular disease. Support from mental health professionals, support groups, or even close friends and family can make a substantial difference in managing emotional challenges.

Lifestyle Modifications: Making necessary lifestyle changes, such as adopting a heart-healthy diet, quitting smoking, and managing stress, can help control risk factors like high blood pressure and reduce the likelihood of further cerebrovascular events.

Assistive Devices and Technology: Advancements in assistive devices and technology have greatly improved the quality of life for individuals with cerebrovascular disease.

These tools can aid in mobility, communication, and daily living tasks.

Finding Hope

Living with cerebrovascular disease can be daunting, but hope can be found in several aspects of this journey:

Medical Advances: Ongoing research and medical advancements continue to improve our understanding of cerebrovascular disease and its treatment options. New therapies, medications, and interventions are continually emerging, offering hope for better outcomes.

Resilience: Many individuals living with cerebrovascular disease demonstrate remarkable resilience. They adapt to challenges, learn new skills, and find ways to live fulfilling lives despite physical limitations.

Supportive Communities: Joining support groups or connecting with others facing similar challenges can provide a sense of belonging and shared experiences. These communities offer a place to exchange advice, share successes, and seek emotional support.

Personal Growth:

Some individuals discover new strengths and facets of their identity as they navigate life with cerebrovascular disease. The journey can lead to personal growth, increased self-awareness, and a deeper appreciation for life's precious moments.

In conclusion, living with cerebrovascular disease is a complex and multifaceted experience that encompasses physical, emotional, and lifestyle challenges. However, with the right support systems, medical care, and a positive mindset, individuals can find hope and live meaningful lives despite the hurdles they face. Advances in medical science and the resilience of the human spirit offer promise for a brighter future for those affected by cerebrovascular disease.

Life after stroke: navigating daily challenges

A stroke, often described as a "brain attack," can be a life-altering event. Survivors and their loved ones face profound changes as they navigate the path to recovery. In this essay, we will explore what life can be like after a stroke, the challenges that come with it, and the resilience and hope that can be found in rebuilding one's life.

The Immediate Impact:

The immediate aftermath of a stroke is often marked by confusion and fear. Survivors may experience physical, cognitive, and emotional challenges. These can include paralysis or weakness on one side of the body, difficulty with speech or communication, memory problems, and emotional upheaval.

Rehabilitation and Recovery:

Rehabilitation is a critical phase of post-stroke life. It involves a combination of physical therapy, occupational therapy, and speech therapy tailored to the individual's needs. This phase can be physically and emotionally demanding, as survivors work tirelessly to regain lost abilities.

Rehabilitation is not only about regaining physical function but also about rebuilding confidence and a sense of self. Many survivors find that their determination and the support of therapists and loved ones help them make significant progress.

Adapting to a New Normal:

Life after a stroke often involves adapting to a new normal. Survivors may need mobility aids like wheelchairs or walkers, assistive devices for daily tasks, and home modifications for accessibility and safety. These adjustments can be challenging, but they are crucial for regaining independence.

Cognitive and Emotional Changes:

Stroke survivors may also grapple with cognitive changes, such as memory deficits or difficulty concentrating. Emotional challenges are common too, including depression and anxiety. These changes can be just as challenging as physical ones and require specialized care and support.

Support Systems:

Having a strong support system is invaluable during the journey of life after stroke. Family, friends, and caregivers play a pivotal role in providing emotional support, assisting with daily tasks, and motivating survivors to keep pushing forward.

Finding Hope and Resilience:

While the challenges of life after stroke are significant, so too are the opportunities for hope and resilience:

- **Recovery Is Possible: Many stroke survivors make remarkable recoveries, regaining lost functions over time. Consistent rehabilitation, determination, and patience can yield substantial improvements.**

- **Embracing New Hobbies and Interests: Life after stroke often leads to the discovery of new passions and interests. Survivors may explore creative pursuits, engage in adaptive sports, or become advocates for stroke awareness.**

- **Support Groups: Connecting with other stroke survivors through support groups can provide a sense of community and understanding. Sharing experiences and strategies for coping can be empowering.**

- **Focus on Prevention:** Many survivors become advocates for stroke prevention, educating others about risk factors and the importance of a healthy lifestyle. This proactive approach can provide a sense of purpose and fulfillment.

- **Quality of Life:** Life after stroke can still be rich and fulfilling. Many survivors find renewed appreciation for life's simple joys and the importance of cherishing the moments that matter.

In conclusion, life after a stroke is a journey marked by change, challenges, and resilience. While the immediate impact can be daunting, with the right support and determination, survivors can rebuild their lives and find hope in the process. Through rehabilitation, adaptation, and the discovery of new passions, life after stroke can be a testament to the human spirit's ability to overcome adversity and embrace a meaningful and fulfilling existence.

Support networks and resources after stroke

A stroke is a life-altering event that can have profound physical, emotional, and psychological impacts on individuals and their families. One of the critical components of stroke recovery is having a strong support network and access to resources. This network of support plays a pivotal role in helping stroke survivors regain their independence, cope with the challenges they face, and improve their overall quality of life.

Immediately after a stroke, the support network often begins with healthcare professionals. Stroke survivors are typically hospitalized, and during this time, they receive care from a team of doctors, nurses, and therapists. This initial phase of recovery is crucial for stabilizing the patient's condition and assessing the extent of the damage. It is also when family members often become key advocates, working closely with medical teams to understand the treatment plan and provide emotional support.

Once the acute phase has passed, stroke survivors often transition to rehabilitation. This is where an even broader support network comes into play. Rehabilitation teams can include physical therapists, occupational therapists, speech therapists, and social workers. These professionals help stroke survivors regain lost abilities, such as mobility, speech, and daily living skills. They also educate patients and their families about stroke recovery and coping strategies.

In addition to healthcare professionals, support often comes from family and friends. The emotional and practical assistance that loved ones provide can be invaluable. Family members may help with tasks like transportation, meal preparation, and household chores. They can also offer emotional support by simply being there to listen, comfort, and encourage the stroke survivor.

Support groups are another critical resource for stroke survivors and their families. These groups provide a sense of community and understanding that can be difficult to find elsewhere. In a support group, individuals can share their experiences, fears, and triumphs with others who have been through similar challenges. This can reduce feelings of isolation and provide valuable insights into coping strategies.

Furthermore, support networks often extend beyond the immediate family and support groups. Many communities have organizations and agencies dedicated to assisting stroke survivors. These organizations may offer educational resources, access to adaptive equipment, and information about financial assistance programs. They can help stroke survivors navigate the complex healthcare system and connect them with valuable resources.

Another essential aspect of stroke recovery is mental health support. Stroke survivors frequently experience depression, anxiety, and other emotional challenges. Mental health professionals, such as psychologists or psychiatrists, can provide therapy and counseling to address these issues. Managing mental health is a crucial part of the overall recovery process.

As time goes on, the support network may evolve as the stroke survivor's needs change. Some individuals may return to work, while others may require ongoing assistance with daily living activities. In either case, the support network remains vital. Workplace accommodations and vocational rehabilitation services can help stroke survivors re-enter the workforce, while home healthcare services can provide assistance with daily tasks.

In conclusion, stroke recovery is a complex and often long-term journey that requires a strong support network and access to various resources. This network includes healthcare professionals, family, friends, support groups, community organizations, and mental health experts. Together, they provide physical, emotional, and practical support to help stroke survivors regain their independence and improve their overall quality of life. Building and maintaining this support network is a crucial aspect of stroke recovery and can make a significant difference in a person's ability to overcome the challenges posed by a stroke.

Chapter 12

Future directions and hopes for stroke

The future directions and hopes for stroke research and treatment are promising, as scientists, healthcare professionals, and technology continue to advance. Stroke, a devastating and often life-altering medical event, affects millions of people worldwide. While strides have been made in prevention and treatment, there is still much work to be done.

One of the most significant hopes for the future of stroke lies in prevention. As our understanding of the risk factors for stroke deepens, there is an opportunity to develop more effective prevention strategies. Lifestyle modifications, such as improved diet and increased physical activity, play a pivotal role in reducing the risk of stroke. Additionally, advancements in genetic research may allow for personalized stroke risk assessments and interventions.

Moreover, the development of novel medical treatments and interventions is a promising avenue. Thrombolytic therapy and mechanical thrombectomy have revolutionized the treatment of acute ischemic strokes. Future research may focus on refining these techniques, making them more widely accessible, and extending their therapeutic window.

Dealing with stroke

Additionally, neuroprotective agents that can limit brain damage following a stroke are actively being investigated, offering hope for improved outcomes.

Telemedicine and remote monitoring technologies are transforming stroke care, particularly in rural or underserved areas. The ability to quickly assess stroke patients and provide expert guidance through telemedicine can significantly reduce treatment delays and improve outcomes. Furthermore, wearable devices and smartphone applications are being developed to monitor vital signs and detect early warning signs of stroke, allowing for timely intervention.

Advancements in neuroimaging are providing insights into the intricacies of stroke and aiding in treatment decisions. Functional MRI and diffusion tensor imaging are helping researchers understand the brain's ability to recover and rewire itself after a stroke. This knowledge may lead to more targeted rehabilitation therapies and a better understanding of individualized recovery trajectories.

In the realm of regenerative medicine, stem cell therapy holds great promise. Stem cells have the potential to repair damaged brain tissue and promote functional recovery in stroke survivors. While this field is still in its infancy, ongoing research and clinical trials are exploring the safety and efficacy of stem cell-based treatments.

Artificial intelligence (AI) and machine learning are playing an increasingly vital role in stroke research and care. These technologies can analyze vast amounts of medical data to predict stroke risk, assist with diagnosis, and optimize treatment plans. AI-powered robotic devices are also being developed to aid in stroke rehabilitation, providing customized exercises and tracking progress.

Furthermore, community education and awareness campaigns are critical components of stroke prevention and early intervention. Public health initiatives aim to educate people about the signs of stroke and the importance of seeking immediate medical attention. By reducing the time between symptom onset and treatment, more stroke patients can benefit from life-saving interventions.

In conclusion, the future of stroke care and research is filled with hope and potential. Advances in prevention, treatment, telemedicine, neuroimaging, regenerative medicine, AI, and public education are collectively working to reduce the devastating impact of strokes on individuals and society. With continued dedication to research and innovation, there is optimism that stroke outcomes will continue to improve, ultimately enhancing the quality of life for stroke survivors and their families.

Innovation in stroke care

Stroke, often referred to as a "brain attack," is a top cause of disfunction and death to millions worldwide. It occurs when there is a sudden disruption of blood supply to the brain, leading to the death of brain cells. While stroke has long been a medical challenge, recent years have witnessed remarkable innovations in both the treatment and prevention of this devastating condition.

Advances in Stroke Treatment

Thrombectomy: One of the most groundbreaking innovations in stroke treatment is the advent of mechanical thrombectomy. This procedure involves the use of a specialized device to physically remove blood clots from blocked arteries in the brain. Thrombectomy has extended the treatment window for stroke patients, allowing many to recover fully when they might have faced severe disability or death in the past.

Telestroke: The integration of telemedicine into stroke care has revolutionized how stroke patients receive treatment. Telestroke enables remote neurologists to assess patients via video conferencing, ensuring rapid access to expert care, especially in underserved rural areas. Timely intervention is critical in stroke management, and telestroke has bridged geographical gaps to improve outcomes.

Neuroimaging: Advanced neuroimaging techniques, such as MRI and CT scans, have improved stroke diagnosis and treatment planning. These technologies provide detailed insights into the brain's condition, helping healthcare professionals identify the type and extent of stroke damage. This precision guides treatment decisions and allows for tailored interventions.

Neuroprotective Therapies: Researchers are exploring innovative neuroprotective strategies to minimize brain damage during a stroke. These therapies aim to preserve brain tissue and reduce the long-term consequences of stroke. Some promising approaches include neuroinflammation modulation and neuroregeneration techniques.

Prevention of Stroke

Targeted Medications: The development of novel medications, such as direct oral anticoagulants (DOACs) and antiplatelet agents, has significantly enhanced stroke prevention. DOACs, in particular, are more convenient and effective than traditional blood thinners like warfarin, reducing the risk of stroke in patients with atrial fibrillation.

Artificial Intelligence (AI): AI-driven algorithms are aiding in stroke risk prediction by analyzing various factors, including medical history, genetic data, and lifestyle choices. These algorithms can identify individuals at high risk of stroke, enabling early interventions such as lifestyle modifications or medication.

Remote Monitoring: Wearable devices and remote monitoring systems have empowered individuals to track their health continuously. For stroke survivors and those at risk, these technologies provide real-time data on vital signs, allowing for early detection of warning signs and immediate medical attention if needed.

Community Education: Innovative outreach programs and digital platforms are educating the public about stroke risk factors and prevention strategies. These initiatives use interactive tools, mobile apps, and social media to engage individuals in managing their health and making informed choices.

Research and Future Directions

Stem Cell Therapy: Ongoing research in stem cell therapy holds potential for regenerating damaged brain tissue after a stroke. Early studies have shown promising results in animal models, sparking hope for future clinical applications.

Genetic Insights: Genetic studies are uncovering new stroke-related genes and pathways, shedding light on personalized prevention and treatment approaches. Understanding an individual's genetic predisposition to stroke could lead to targeted interventions.

Brain-Computer Interfaces (BCIs): BCIs are being explored for stroke rehabilitation. These devices allow direct communication between the brain and external devices, offering new avenues for patients to regain motor and cognitive functions.

Nutritional Innovation: The role of diet in stroke prevention is continuously evolving. Innovations in personalized nutrition plans and functional foods tailored to individual health profiles may prove instrumental in reducing stroke risk.

In conclusion, innovation in stroke care has transformed the landscape of both treatment and prevention. Advances in thrombectomy, telemedicine, neuroimaging, and neuroprotective therapies have revolutionized stroke treatment. Meanwhile, targeted medications, AI-driven risk prediction, remote monitoring, and community education have improved stroke prevention. As research continues to push boundaries in areas like stem cell therapy, genetics, BCIs, and nutrition, the outlook for stroke patients and those at risk is increasingly hopeful. Stroke, once considered a dire medical emergency with limited options, is now a field of pioneering innovation with the potential to save lives and improve outcomes on a global scale.

Rehabilitation on stroke care

Stroke is a devastating medical condition that affects millions of individuals worldwide, causing significant disability and often requiring extensive rehabilitation. Stroke rehabilitation is a critical component of recovery, aimed at improving the physical, cognitive, and emotional well-being of stroke survivors. In this story we will explore the key aspects of stroke rehabilitation, including its goals, approaches, and the multidisciplinary team involved in the process.

Understanding Stroke

Before delving into rehabilitation, it's essential to understand stroke itself. Stroke occurs when there is a disruption in the supply of blood to the brain. This disruption can be due to a blocked blood vessel (ischemic stroke) or a ruptured blood vessel (hemorrhagic stroke). The brain cells deprived of oxygen and nutrients begin to die, leading to various impairments, including paralysis, speech difficulties, and cognitive deficits.

Goals of Stroke Rehabilitation

Stroke rehabilitation has several primary goals, which can be summarized as follows:

- Maximizing Functional Independence: One of the primary objectives of stroke rehabilitation is to help individuals regain as much independence as possible in their daily activities. This includes improving mobility, self-care skills, and the ability to perform routine tasks.

- Preventing Complications: Stroke survivors are at risk of developing complications like muscle contractures, pressure sores, and pneumonia due to reduced mobility. Rehabilitation aims to minimize these risks.

135

- **Improving Communication:** Many stroke survivors experience aphasia, a language impairment that affects their ability to communicate. Speech therapy is a vital component of rehabilitation to help individuals regain their ability to speak and understand language.

- **Enhancing Cognitive Function:** Stroke can impact cognitive functions such as memory, attention, and problem-solving. Rehabilitation may include cognitive therapy to address these issues.

Multidisciplinary Approach

Stroke rehabilitation is not a one-size-fits-all process. It requires a multidisciplinary team of healthcare professionals who collaborate to provide comprehensive care tailored to the individual's needs. Here are some key members of the rehabilitation team:

Physical Therapists: They focus on improving mobility, strength, and balance. Exercises and techniques are used to help stroke survivors regain the ability to walk and perform other physical tasks.

Occupational Therapists: These professionals work on improving the skills needed for daily living, such as dressing, cooking, and bathing. They help stroke survivors regain independence in these essential activities.

Speech Therapists: Speech therapists, or speech-language pathologists, help individuals recover their ability to speak, understand language, and swallow safely.

Neuropsychologists: These specialists assess and treat cognitive impairments. They work on memory, attention, and problem-solving skills to enhance overall cognitive function.

Social Workers: Stroke survivors and their families often face significant social and emotional challenges. Social workers provide support, connect families with resources, and address psychosocial needs.

Nurses: Nurses play a crucial role in managing medical needs, preventing complications, and providing ongoing care and education to both patients and their families.

Recreational Therapists: They use recreational activities as a means of rehabilitation, aiming to improve physical, emotional, and social well-being.

Nutritionists: Proper nutrition is essential for recovery. Nutritionists assess dietary needs and provide guidance to ensure stroke survivors receive the necessary nutrients for healing.

Caregivers and Family: Family members often serve as primary caregivers and play an indispensable role in the rehabilitation process. They may receive training and support to assist in care.

Challenges in Stroke Rehabilitation

Stroke rehabilitation can be a lengthy and challenging process. Progress varies widely among individuals, and some may experience frustration or setbacks. Additionally, access to rehabilitation services can be limited in certain regions, leading to disparities in care.

In recent years, technological advancements have played a significant role in stroke rehabilitation. Virtual reality, robotics, and telemedicine have expanded the possibilities for remote monitoring and therapy, potentially improving access to care.

In conclusion, stroke rehabilitation is a complex and multifaceted process aimed at helping individuals regain independence and improve their quality of life after a stroke. It involves a team of healthcare professionals working together to address physical, cognitive, and emotional challenges. While challenges exist, ongoing research and technological advancements continue to enhance the effectiveness of stroke rehabilitation, offering hope and improved outcomes for stroke survivors.

The path forward(improving stroke outcome)

Stroke, a sudden disruption of blood supply to the brain, is a leading cause of disability and death worldwide. While medical advances have significantly improved our understanding and treatment of strokes, there remains a pressing need to further enhance outcomes for stroke patients. The path forward to improving stroke outcomes involves a multifaceted approach encompassing prevention, acute care, rehabilitation, and ongoing support.

1. Prevention is Paramount

The first step on the path to improving stroke outcomes is prevention. Stroke risk factors, such as high blood pressure, smoking, obesity, and diabetes, are well-established. Public health campaigns must continue to educate the public on these risk factors and promote healthy lifestyle choices. Government policies can play a crucial role in reducing these risk factors through measures like tobacco taxes and improved access to healthy foods.

Furthermore, early detection of conditions that increase stroke risk, like atrial fibrillation, should be a priority. The development and adoption of affordable and non-invasive screening technologies can help identify at-risk individuals, allowing for timely intervention.

2. Revolutionizing Acute Care

The acute care phase following a stroke is critical, and advancements in this area have the potential to significantly impact outcomes. Telemedicine and remote monitoring technologies have gained prominence, enabling faster access to expert stroke care, especially in rural or underserved areas. Telestroke programs connect remote physicians with specialized stroke centers, allowing for rapid evaluation and treatment decisions.

In addition to telemedicine, advancements in imaging techniques and artificial intelligence (AI) have transformed stroke diagnosis and treatment. AI algorithms can analyze brain images to identify stroke patterns quickly, aiding in the timely administration of clot-busting medications like tissue plasminogen activator (tPA) or thrombectomy procedures.

Moreover, research into neuroprotective agents that minimize brain damage during a stroke is ongoing. New pharmaceuticals and therapies that reduce inflammation and oxidative stress may enhance the brain's resilience to ischemia.

3. Personalized Rehabilitation

Recovery after a stroke is a challenging journey, and personalized rehabilitation is key to improving outcomes. Advances in neurorehabilitation techniques, including robotics and virtual reality, offer tailored therapy programs that cater to the specific needs of each patient. These technologies can engage patients in more interactive and motivating exercises, potentially speeding up recovery.

Furthermore, tele-rehabilitation can extend access to post-stroke therapy for those who may have difficulty traveling to rehabilitation centers. Through video conferencing and wearable devices, therapists can guide and monitor patients remotely, ensuring consistent progress.

4. Long-Term Support and Secondary Prevention

The path to improved stroke outcomes extends far beyond the acute phase and initial rehabilitation. Providing ongoing support and secondary prevention strategies are crucial components. Support groups and community-based programs can help stroke survivors and their families cope with the emotional and physical challenges that arise post-stroke.

Secondary prevention, such as the management of risk factors like hypertension and diabetes, should be a lifelong commitment. Health systems should implement robust follow-up care and monitoring to prevent recurrent strokes. Medication adherence programs and regular check-ups can play a pivotal role in maintaining optimal health.

5. Advancing Research and Innovation

Research is the engine that propels progress in stroke care. Continued investment in stroke research is essential to uncovering novel treatments and interventions. Collaborative efforts between academia, healthcare institutions, and the pharmaceutical industry can accelerate the development of new therapies.

Furthermore, exploring the genetic and molecular underpinnings of stroke susceptibility can lead to personalized medicine approaches. Identifying genetic markers associated with stroke risk can help tailor prevention and treatment strategies to an individual's unique genetic profile.

6. Enhancing Stroke Education

Education is the cornerstone of stroke prevention and improvement of outcomes. Public awareness campaigns must persistently communicate the signs and symptoms of stroke, emphasizing the importance of seeking immediate medical attention. Schools, workplaces, and communities can also play a role in teaching basic life support and stroke recognition skills.

Moreover, healthcare providers should receive ongoing training in the latest stroke treatment protocols and technologies. Continuous medical education ensures that stroke patients receive the best possible care.

7. Global Collaboration

Stroke knows no borders, and global collaboration is vital for advancing stroke care worldwide. Sharing best practices, research findings, and resources can help developing nations improve their stroke infrastructure. International organizations and governments can work together to create a global framework for stroke prevention, treatment, and research.

In conclusion, the path forward to improving stroke outcomes is paved with a combination of prevention, acute care advancements, personalized rehabilitation, long-term support, ongoing research, education, and global collaboration. By addressing stroke comprehensively and holistically, we can aspire to reduce the devastating impact of stroke on individuals and communities, offering hope and a brighter future to those affected by this condition.